Advances in Experimental Medicine and Biology

Volume 1151

More information about this series at http://www.springer.com/series/5584

Federico Garrido

MHC Class-I Loss and Cancer Immune Escape

Springer

Federico Garrido
Departamento de Analisis Clinicos e Inmunologia,
Hospital Universitario Virgen de las Nieves,
Facultad de Medicina
Universidad de Granada
Granada, Spain

ISSN 0065-2598 ISSN 2214-8019 (electronic)
Advances in Experimental Medicine and Biology
ISBN 978-3-030-17863-5 ISBN 978-3-030-17864-2 (eBook)
https://doi.org/10.1007/978-3-030-17864-2

This Springer imprint is published by the registered company Springer Nature Switzerland AG.
The registered company address is: Gewerbestrasse 11, 6330 Cham, Switzerland

Acknowledgments

The work presented in this book summarizes decades of research focused on analyzing the expression of histocompatibility antigens in mouse and human tumors (H-2 and HLA) in the Dept. of Analisis Clinicos e Inmunologia at Hospital Universitario "Virgen de las Nieves" in Granada, Spain. I would like to acknowledge all the members of the research team for their contributions. Most importantly, I would like to thank the cancer patients in our hospital and from different European clinical and research institutions who gave their consent to analyze their tumor samples. I would like to mention Dr. Matias Perez who started to work with me in 1979 and initiated the mouse work at the beginning of the 1980s by inducing experimental sarcomas with methylcholanthrene and typing different tumor clones for H-2 antigens. One of these tumors, the GR9, and all the different tumor clones obtained have been studied for more than 20 years by him and other researchers in our group, Ignacio Algarra, Jose Juan Gaforio, and Angel Garcia Lora. These studies have generated important discoveries. We have learned a lot and are still obtaining new data from the GR9 tumor model. Dr. Teresa Cabrera set up the immunohistological laboratory and developed tumor microdissection techniques to study HLA expression in human tumor tissues. She selected a large variety of monoclonal antibodies that recognize different HLA antigens in tumor tissues and participated in the International HLA workshop in France where the "HLA and cancer" component was introduced for the first time. Dr. Francisco Ruiz-Cabello applied different molecular and flow cytometry techniques to identify and characterize molecular mechanisms responsible for HLA alterations. He and his team, including Drs. Pilar Jimenez and Isabel Maleno, made important contributions to the field. Dr. Miguel Angel Lopez-Nevot in the early days focused on melanoma and on genomic HLA typing of tumors, helping to develop the immunofluorescence techniques with anti-HLA monoclonal antibodies. Dr. Natalia Aptsiauri brought her enormous international experience to our team, which she had gained from different USA labs, and collaborated with me in writing different reviews and taking strategic decisions in our work. All of them currently are holding important academic and research positions at the University of Granada and Jaen, as well as in the Tumour Tissue Biobank of the Hospital Universitario Virgen de las Nieves.

I also would like to thank clinical collaborators from our University Hospital, including Dr. Angel Concha, the head of the Pathology Dept. who was directly involved in providing cryopreserved tumor tissues of different origin, for the productive cooperation that we have had for many years in difficult times; Dr. Miguel Tallada and Dr. Jose Manuel Cozar (Urology Dept.), Drs. Antonio Cueto and Abel Sanchez-Palencia (Thoracic Surgery), Dr. Javier Gutierrez and Dr. Antonio Ferron (General Surgery), Prof. Francisco Esteban and Dr. Jose Salinero (Otorhinolaryngology Dept.), Prof. Alfonso Herruzo (Gynecology Dept.), and Prof. Salvio Serrano (Dermatology), for cooperating with us at different time periods providing fresh tumor tissue samples of different origin; and the pathologist Dr. Miguel Angel Piris from Madrid and the immunologists Dr. Francisco Real and Prof. Miguel Lopez-Botet from Barcelona for helping to design new approaches in the HLA and cancer field.

I must also mention important and diverse international cooperations that we developed over the years starting with the collaboration with Dr. Peter Stern from the Patterson Institute in Manchester, England. We published two highly quoted reviews in 1993 and 1997, which summarize the work carried out in Granada and Manchester in the 1980s and 1990s in relation to HLA expression in human tumors. Dr. Eva Klein from the Karolinska Institute has been interested in this area of research from the very beginning and organized, together with Dr. Hilliard Festenstein from the London Hospital, the first meeting on "Histocompatibility Antigens in Tumors" that took place in Granada in 1985 (see J of Immunogenetics Vol.13, n°2/3, 1986). Drs. Klass Karre and Hans-Gustaf Ljunggren from the same institution collaborated with us in defining the complexity of the different clones of the mouse GR9 fibrosarcoma. Dr. Soldano Ferrone, a pioneer in the HLA and cancer field, collaborated with us when he was working in New York State, in Pittsburg, and later in Harvard University in Boston. Dr. Francesco Marincola at the NIH (USA) helped us to analyze in detail progressing and regressing metastatic lesions in mixed responder melanoma patients. Together with Dr. Marcel Tilanus and Manita Feenstra from Utrecht, we developed novel techniques to define HLA haplotype losses in human tumors and participated in the HLA workshops. With another leading scientist in our field, Dr. Barbara Seliger from Halle in Germany, we collaborated in the investigations of "the antigen presentation machinery" in tumor cells. I have to mention an important collaboration with Drs. Dirk Schadendorf and Annette Paschen (Mannhein and Essen) in defining new molecular mechanisms responsible for HLA alterations in melanoma. With Dr. Gustav Gaudernak and his team at the Norwegian Radium Hospital in Oslo, we have a long-term collaboration studying HLA class I loss in tumor immune escape and cancer progression. Dr. Thierry Boon and Pierre Coulie from the Ludwig Institute in Brussels, who pioneered the identification of tumor antigens recognized by T lymphocytes, cooperated with us in defining HLA-I-associated tumor immune escape mechanisms in patients receiving peptide immunotherapy. With Drs. Alex Knuth (Mainz), Catia Traversari (Milan), and Jesper Zeuthen (Copenhagen), we worked closely defining new molecular mechanisms of HLA alteration in melanoma. With Drs. Graham Pawelec (Tubingen) and Steve Marsh (London), we collaborated in an EU project in which a European melanoma cell bank (ESTADB) has been developed.

I want to highlight the period I spent as a postdoctoral fellow in the London Hospital Medical College under the supervision of Dr. Hilliard Festenstein.

He helped me to start a new project in his lab typing H-2 antigens in mouse tumors in 1974–1975. I learned immunogenetics of the H-2 system and applied this knowledge to the altered HLA expression observed in tumor cells. This was the beginning of my journey in the field of "MHC and cancer." Drs. Dominique Charron (Paris) and Renee Fauchet (Nantes) introduced for the first time the "HLA and cancer" component in the XII International Histocompatibility workshop in 1996. I would also like to thank the Spanish Medical Research Council (Fondo de Investigaciones Sanitarias, FIS) for financing our research since 1981 and "Ramon Areces Foundation" in Spain for financing the "HLA and Cancer" meetings organized in Granada in 1998 and 2011. I would like to thank many different PhD and postdoctoral students that worked in our group at Hospital Universitario Virgen de las Nieves in Granada since 1981: Javier Martin, Concha Delgado, Rosario Oliva, Susana Pedrinaci, Maria Luisa Garrido, Antonio Garrido, Abelardo Caballero, Maximino Redondo, Julia Canton, Alfonso Serrano, Rosa Mendez, Jose Maria Romero, Monica Bernal, Teresa Rodriguez, Francisco Perea, Luis Miguel Real, Rafael and Javier Carretero, Irene Romero, Cristina Garrido, Ana Belen del Campo, Isabel Maleno, and Greta Garrido from the Molecular Immunology Institute of Havana, Cuba. All made important discoveries published in leading international journals. I would specifically thank Dr. Monica Bernal for her help in making different figures of this book, Dr. Fran Perea for the images of tissue immunohistochemistry, Dr. Teresa Rodriguez and Maria Jose Olivares for helping me with the reference list, and Drs. Natalia Aptsiauri, Francisco Ruiz-Cabello, and Angel Garcia Lora for the critical review of the book. Finally, I would like to thank my family, my wife, Antonia Collado, who has been always by my side in difficult moments and helped me with my research for many years working in the Research Unit of our Hospital, and my three daughters, Pilar, Carolina, and Nona, who missed me many times when I was travelling to different places and meetings.

This book summarizes the progress made in the field of "MHC and Cancer Immune Escape" and the contributions made by many scientists all over the world. Nevertheless, there is still a long way before we fully understand the "stealth technology" used by cancer cells to escape and find new methods to fight it that can be applied in the clinic. MHC was discovered in experiments with tumor transplantation in mice. The impact of HLA tissue typing in human transplantation helped to improve our knowledge about this complex genetic system. Now MHC/HLA returns to cancer owing its important role in tumor rejection and escape. The MHC system did not evolve to fight cancer but is no doubt playing a pivotal role. Perhaps, MHC is now "repaying" to cancer cells for being discovered. It is likely that "MHC and cancer" will be travelling together for the years to come.

Contents

Introduction

1

Abstract

This chapter focuses on the discovery of the Major Histocompatibility Complex (MHC) in mice (H-2) and in humans (HLA), and on the role played by the International HLA Workshops in the analysis and characterization of this complex genetic system. The early days of Tumour Immunology and the importance of the definition of Tumour Associated Transplantation Antigens (TATA) are also discussed. Today we know that tumour cells can be killed by T lymphocytes by recognizing tumour antigenic peptides presented by MHC molecules and they can also escape this recognition by losing the expression of MHC molecules. This important phenomenon has been profoundly studied for many years both in my lab in Granada and in other laboratories. The results of this research have important implications for the new generation of cancer immunotherapy that boosts T cell responses. A historical perspective of major discoveries is presented in this chapter, with the names of the scientists that have made a significant contribution to the enormous progress made in the field of Tumour Immunology.

Keywords

MHC · HLA · H-2 · Major histocompatibility complex · HLA heavy chain · Beta2 microglobulin · Tumor immunology · Tumor escape · HLA workshops · Antigen processing

Peter Gorer discovered the Histocompatibility system (H-2) in mice in 1935 in experiments with allogeneic tumor transplantation. The key observation was that tumors fail to growth when transplanted into genetically distinct host of the same species. The antibodies generated in these alloimmunizations were used for MHC typing of red blood cells in inbred strains of mice using a complement-dependent cytotoxicity test (Gorer 1936, 1937; Gorer and Mikulska 1954; Gorer and O'Gorman 1956). This test was used years later to discover and define the HLA system in humans by testing leukocytes with alloimmune sera obtained from individuals after blood transfusion (Dausset 1954) and from pregnant women (van Rood 1962). I recommend reading the article "*Seeds of time: Fifty years ago Peter A. Gorer discovered the H-2 complex*" written by Jean Klein (1986), the publication by Bernard Amos on "*Recollections of Dr Peter Gorer*" (1986) and the book "*H-2 antigens: genes, molecules, function*" edited by Shella David (1987) after the meeting he organized in the Jackson Lab in Bar Harbor (Maine, USA) to commemorate the 50th anniversary of the discovery of the H-2 system (see also Snell 1986).

In 1975–1976 mouse tumors were typed for H-2 antigens in the laboratory of Hilliard Festenstein at the London Hospital Medical College using mouse alloantisera, defining private and public H-2 specificities (Garrido et al. 1976, 1977, 1979; Schmidt et al. 1979). The key finding was that the MHC class I profiles

F. Garrido, *MHC Class-I Loss and Cancer Immune Escape*, Advances in Experimental Medicine and Biology 1151, https://doi.org/10.1007/978-3-030-17864-2_1

obtained when typing mouse tumors were not the same as those corresponding to autologous/syngeneic lymphoid cells. Extra reactivities as well as the absense of expected reactions (H-2 class I losses) were discovered. The former were, most likely, due to the anti-viral antibodies present in the mouse alloantisera. The latter were unexpected H-2 reactivity patterns that could not be clearly explained at the time. This work was the beginning of a history with important implications in Tumour Immunology and Clinical Oncology (Festenstein and Schmidt 1981; Festenstein 1987).

HLA tumor typing in human melanoma and colorectal carcinoma was performed in the 80s in tumor tissues using anti-HLA monoclonal antibodies that recognize monomorphic determinants (Ruiter et al. 1982; Natali et al. 1983; Csiba et al. 1984). The HLA class I positive staining of the tumor stroma was always used as an internal control (Ruiter et al. 1984, 1986; Natali et al. 1984; Lopez-Nevot et al. 1986; Moore et al. 1986; Cabrera et al. 2003). It was evident from the very beginning that HLA typing of tumor tissues did not match that of autologous peripheral blood lymphocytes of a particular cancer patient. The absence of HLA class I expression was detected with anti-HLA MoAbs directed against common HLA A,B,C determinants, against the β2 microglobulin or against particular HLA class I alleles (Lopez-Nevot et al. 1989; Natali et al. 1989). After decades of research doing HLA typing of tumor tissues by different groups including ourselves, it has become accepted that altered tumor HLA class I expression is a major finding due to its high frequency and its relevance in cancer immune escape (Garrido et al. 1993; Marincola et al. 2000; Garrido and Algarra 2001).

There is strong evidence suggesting that HLA class I cell surface expression in tumor cells plays a pivotal role in the recognition and destruction of nascent tumors due to its role in antigen presentation to T lymphocytes. Loss or downregulation of MHC/HLA class I molecules is a key mechanism used by tumor cells to escape from T cell responses, as it has been demonstrated by different research groups (Schmidt and Festenstein 1982; Festenstein and Garrido 1986; Smith et al. 1989; Bodmer et al. 1993; Garrido et al. 1995; Ruiz-Cabello and Garrido 2002). Viruses also use similar escape strategies (Schrier et al. 1983; Alcami and Koszinowski 2000). Although this mechanism was described in mouse and human tumors many years ago (Garrido et al. 1979, 1997; Festenstein 1987; Garrido and Klein 1991; Marincola et al. 2000), it has been ignored for decades. However, a revival of the topic "*HLA and cancer immune escape*" is now in progress with new reports by different groups involving HLA in tumor escape (Lampen and van Hall 2011; Chowell et al. 2017; McGranahan et al. 2017; Sucker et al. 2017; Grasso et al. 2018; Aptsiauri et al. 2018). The old idea that the immune system is capable to constantly survey and destroy transformed cells in our body (Burnet 1957, 1970, 1971; Thomas 1959) was confirmed when a particular tumor escape mechanism had been defined in a given tumor (Villunger and Strasser 1999).

This book analyzes the relevance of MHC/HLA expression for the immune escape in primary tumors and metastasis, including experimental data obtained in chemically induced sarcomas, as well as in human tumors. These data are the result of many years of work in the Clinical Laboratory of the "*Hospital Universitario Virgen de las Nieves*" in Granada, Spain. During this long period of time, which started in the late 70s, five scientific meetings took place in Granada (Spain) on the topic "HLA and Cancer". The first one was held in 1985 with the title: "*Histocompatibility Antigens on Tumours*". A special issue of the Journal of Immunogenetics published a set of papers on this topic presented during the meeting (see Butcher G, Journal of Immunogenetics 1986 Vol 13, N° 2/3, April/June). The second one took place in 1991 and was titled: "*MHC molecules in normal and neoplastic cells*". A special issue of the International Journal of Cancer reported the different presentations that took place at the meeting (see Garrido F, Int J Cancer 1991, supplement 6). The third one in 1994 in the city of Jaen, near Granada with the title of "*Oncogenes, tumour antigens and MHC Molecules*" and reported in volume 47 of Tissue Antigens 1996 (see Garrido 1996). The fourth one took place in 1998 in

Granada with the title of: "*Tumour Antigens and MHC molecules: Mechanism of tumour escape from the immune system, implications for immunotherapy*" and the last one in the village of Dílar near by Granada in October, 2011 with the title of "*Cancer Immune escape: implications for immunotherapy*" (Aptsiauri et al. 2012). Also the PIVAC 6 meeting (Progress in Vaccination Against Cancer) was organized in our hospital in Granada in 2006 and was dedicated to HLA and Cancer (Aptsiauri et al. 2007a). The Granada meetings in Tumour Immunology had a common goal, namely, to analyze the role of MHC antigens in cancer immune escape.

1.1 The Early Days of Tumour Immunology

The ability of the immune system to reject tumors in syngeneic animals was first demonstrated in inbred mice with chemically induced sarcomas (Gross 1943; Foley 1953; Baldwin 1955; Prehn and Main 1957; Klein et al. 1960). Mice immunized with a particular sarcoma were protected against the same tumor but not against other types. These experiments, done in different labs during the last century, originated the concept of "*Tumour Associated Transplantation Antigens*" (TATA) and also introduced the idea of "*Individual-Unique Tumour Antigens*" (Basombrio 1970). These discoveries were in line with the idea proposed at the time by McFarlane Burnet that the immune system can survey the cells of our body. He wrote: "*It is an evolutionary necessity that there should be some mechanism for eliminating or inactivating such potentially dangerous mutant cells and it is postulated that this mechanism is of immunological character*" (Burnet 1957, 1970, 1971). A major breakthrough in immunology was the discovery that T lymphocyte-mediated cytotoxicity (CTL) is restricted by MHC molecules (Zinkernagel and Doherty 1974, 1979, 1997; Zinkernagel 1996) and that virus antigens are recognized as small peptides inside the structure of the MHC molecules (Bjorkman et al. 1987; Townsend et al. 1986).

The discovery of NK cells by Rolf Kiessling and colleagues at the Tumor Biology Department of the Karolinska Institute (Kiessling et al. 1975; Kiessling and Wigzell 1979) opened a new field also associated with MHC-I/HLA-I cell surface expression in tumors and virus infected cells. Several years later in the same Department it was reported that NK cells are activated by the "*absence*" of MHC class I molecules in the tumor target, raising the provocative idea of the "*Missing Self hypothesis*" with important implications in Tumor Immunology (Kärre et al. 1986; Ljunggren and Kärre 1986, 1990; Kärre 1997). The discovery of tumor antigens recognized by T lymphocytes was also an important accomplishment made at the Ludwig Institute in Brussels by Thierry Boon and colleagues (Boon 1983; Van der Bruggen et al. 1991; Boon et al. 1994, 1996, 2006). They showed that "shared or unique-mutated tumor peptides" are recognized by T lymphocytes and restricted by the expression of a particular MHC/HLA-I allele. The expression of the MAGE genes in melanoma and other tumors were extensively tested for T cell responses recognizing the corresponding tumor peptides presented by different HLA class I alleles (Chomez et al. 2001). All these findings clearly indicated that MHC/HLA molecules play a crucial role in immune responses against viral infections and cancer by interacting with T and NK cell receptors.

Historically, the main objective of cancer immunotherapy has been boosting T cell responses against tumors. This includes BCG therapy in superficial bladder cancer (Morales et al. 1976), Interleukin-2 (Rosenberg et al. 1987), immunization with tumor peptides as tumor antigens (Marchand et al. 1999), dendritic cells loaded with tumor peptides (Nestle et al. 1998), the use of biological response modifiers such as Polysacharide K (PSK) (Nakazato et al. 1994; Nio et al. 1991) and adoptive cell transfer (ACT) using in vitro expanded tumor infiltrating lymphocytes (TIL) in metastatic melanoma (Rosenberg et al. 2011; Andersen et al. 2016). Today cancer immunotherapy is reaching a peak with novel therapies using antibodies that target molecules involved in the regulation of T cell cytotoxicity (Allison et al. 1982, 1995; Leach et al. 1996; Kvistborg et al. 2014; Buferne et al. 2015) reinforcing the idea that T lymphocytes are playing a major role in recognizing and destroying cancer cells (Svane et al. 1999; Boesen et al. 2000; Romero and Coulie 2014). However, only a proportion of cancer patients benefit from this therapy and demonstrate tumor regression, while others develop therapy-resistant progressing metastatic tumor lesions. The reason and underlying mechanisms of these clinical variations are not known. Hence, it is very important to define in the future studies the different escape strategies used in primary and metastatic tumor lesions and personalized suitable therapy in each patient. It is becoming evident that tumors can be rejected, escape or be kept in the state of immune mediated "equilibrium or dormancy", as it was proposed by Bob Schreiber in the "immunoediting" concept (Dunn et al. 2002, 2004). These different tumor/host interactions are very much related to the level of MHC/HLA antigens expressed by the tumor cells (Aptsiauri et al. 2007b; Garrido et al. 2016). Modern cancer immunotherapy will need to monitor the HLA expression levels in tumor tissues in order to avoid ineffective therapies mediated by T cells when the target peptide antigen is not present (Aptsiauri et al. 2008; Thor Straten and Garrido 2016).

1.2 The Major Histocompatibility Complex (MHC): The HLA and the H-2 System

The MHC molecules in humans are called Human Leucocyte Antigens (HLA). The HLA molecules were discovered by alloimmune interactions but they play a major role in antigen presentation to T lymphocytes and in cancer immune escape. It is therefore necessary to briefly summarize our current knowledge about the structure and function of HLA genes and molecules that are expressed in most nucleated cell. Jean Dausset in Paris and JJ Van Rood in Leiden discovered the HLA system (Dausset 1958; van Rood 1962). The 1st International HLA Workshop was organized by Bernard Amos at Duke University in USA in 1964 to exchange anti-HLA sera and to analyze the different reactivities obtained from testing the alloimmune sera against leucocytes using a complement-mediated cytotoxicity test. It was followed by a series of workshops that were organized by pioneers in the HLA field: in 1965 John Van Rood in Leiden (Holland), in 1967 Rugero Cepellini in Torino (Italy), in 1970 Paul Terasaky in Los Angeles (USA), in 1972 Jean Dausset in Paris (France), in 1973 Kisseyer Nielsen in Aarhus (Denmark), in 1977 Walter Bodmer in Oxford (England) and many more, as an example of an International cooperation between scientists to define and understand the structure and function of such a complex biological system. A single laboratory was not able to analyze the multiple different reactivities obtained with many different sera that were tested againts a large variety of leucocytes as targets. It was necessary to exchange these reagents and to compare the patterns of reactivities by different HLA labs. These workshops still take place and the last one was in Standford University (CA, USA) in October 2017, and was organized by Marcelo Fernandez-Viña and Peter Parham. In order to understand the history of HLA and the pioneers that organized such HLA workshops, I recommend reading the Introduction of the 13th International HLA workshop report written by John Hansen (2006) that took place in Victoria (British Columbia) and in Seattle (USA) in 2002. Interestingly, the organization of the HLA workshops was used years later to prepare the Leucocyte Differentiation Antigens workshops that produced the definition of the different molecules called "Clusters of Differentiation" or "CDs" also with an enormous impact in Haematology, Pathology and Clinical Medicine. The first CD Workshop took place in Paris in 1982 and was organized by Alain Bernard; the second one in Boston was organized by Stuart Schlossman, and the third one in Oxford by Andrew McMichael in September of 1986. I recommend reading the introductory remarks of the third CD workshop writen by Cesar Milstein (1987).

Today we know that the HLA system is a complex genetic structure located in the short arm of chromosome six composed of different loci classified in Class I, class II and class III. See review written by Jan Klein in 2000 where this classification was proposed for the first time (Klein and Sato 2000a, b). HLA genes are inherited in a Mendelian form giving rise to the most polymorphic antigenic system that exists in humans (see Fig. 1.1). Within the class I region there are three classical genes (HLA-A, B and C) and three non-classical genes (HLA-E, F, G). Each individual has a combination of six HLA-I classical HLA-I genes (loci A, B and C) in the majority of their cells. The number of HLA-I alleles in the human population is extremely high with 13,262 for HLA class I and 4,846 for HLA class II as defined today. See IPD-IMGT/HLA Database web site for updated details https://www.ebi.ac.uk/ipd/imgt/hla/stats.html.

HLA class I molecules are cell surface glycoproteins composed of highly polymorphic heavy chains encoded by genes located in the short arm of chromosome 6 covalently linked to a constant small molecule i.e. the β2 microglobulin encoded in chromosome 15 (Fig. 1.1). The extracellular part of the heavy chain is devided into three domains: α1, α2 and α3. The peptide binding groove is formed by folding the α1 and α2 domains to create a cleft where the aminoacid

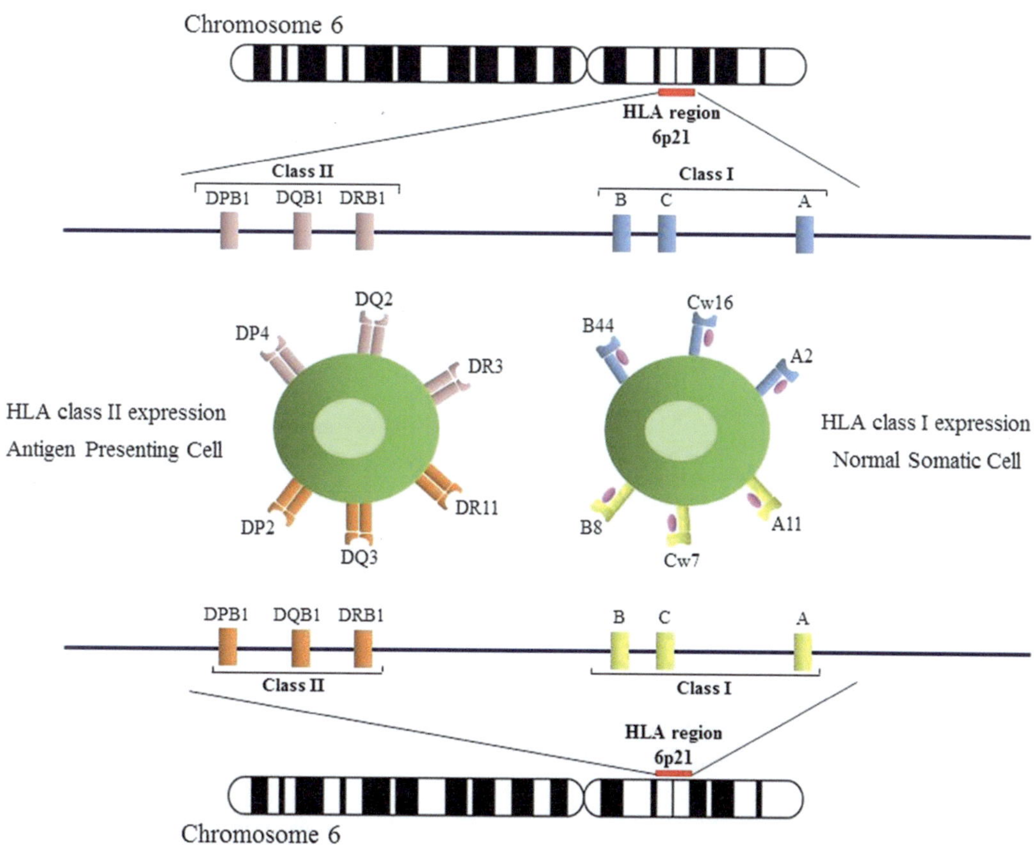

Fig. 1.1 Genetic structure of the Major Histocompatibility Complex in humans (The HLA system) and cell surface expression of HLA I and II molecules. It is located in the 6p21 region of chromosome 6. Any somatic cell expresses six HLA class I alleles composed of a polymorphic heavy chain (A,B,C) and a constant light chain (β2 microglobulin) encoded in chromosome 15. Antigen presenting cells (APCs) express additional 6 HLA class II molecules: DR, DP and DQ composed of two chains (α and β chains) encoded by the genes within the HLA region

Table 1.1 Tissue distribution of HLA class I and II antigens in normal tissues

Tissue	Immunolabeling		Tissue	Inmunolabeling	
	HLA-I	HLA-II		HLA-I	HLA-II
Cells of the endocrine system:			**Urogenital System:**		
Thyroid (follicular, para follicular)	+	–	Kidney glomeruli	++	++
Pancreatic isles of Langerhans	+	–	Kidney tubules	++	++/–/+/–
Grastrointestinal tract:			Epithelium		
Esophagus	++	–	Ureter	++	–
Stomach	+	–	Bladder	++	–
Duodenum	++	++	Prostate	++	–
Colon	++	–	Urethra	++	++
Rectum	++	–	Testis		
Gall bladder	+	ND	Germ cell line, spermatozoa	+	–
Liver			**Miscellaneous:**		
Hepatocytes	+/–	–	Breast epithelium		
Biliary apithelium	++	–/+/–	Ductal	++	++
Respiratory and cardiovascular systems:			Glandular	++	++
Tonsillary epithelium	++	++	**Pancreas**		
Lung (bronchial and alveolar epithelium)	++	ND	Exocrine portion	–	–
Heart			Ductal epitelium	++	–
Myocardium	+	–	**Muscle**		
Endothelium			Skeletal	+/–	–
Capillaries	++	++	Smooth	+	–
Large vessels	++	+/–/+/–	**Langerhans cells, interstitial dentritic cells**	++	++
Nervous system			**Lymphatics**	++	++
Peripheral	++	–	**Fibroblasts**	++	–
Central			**Placenta-villous trophoblas**	–	–
Neurones	–	–	**Epidermis**	+	–

(–) negative; (–/+)…… (+) weakly positive; (++) strongly positive

residues cluster in the hypervariable region (Stern and Wiley 1994). The groove formed by these domains anchor the peptide recognized by the T cell receptor (TCR). Similarly, HLA class II molecules are composed of two polymorphic chains coded by genes located in the centromeric part of the HLA complex and composed of three different loci: HLA DR, DP and DQ (see Fig. 1.1).

Most nucleated cell in the body express six different HLA class I molecules: two HLA-A, two HLA-B and two HLA-C, but the amount of these molecules expressed at the cell surface vary significantly depending on the level of gene transcription, transduction and epigenetic regulation. For instance: normal lymphoid cells are expressing high amount of HLA-I, hepatocytes have lower expression and colorectal normal tissues have an intermediate level. See Table 1.1 summarizing the level of HLA expression in different human tissues. A careful analysis of HLA-I expression in different normal tissues is mandatory since the data that exist were published long time ago using only immunohistological techniques (Daar et al. 1984a). HLA-II molecules have a restricted tissue distribution since are expressed in antigen presenting cells (APCs) such as dendritic cells, macrophages, B cells, activated T lymphocytes and some epithelia, such as cervical and colorectal that are under exogenous exposure to pathogens (Daar et al. 1984b; Cabrera et al. 1995).

HLA class I and II molecules have important immunological functions: the presentation of foreing or altered antigens to T lymphocytes as small peptides inside the HLA structure. Each HLA allele binds and presents to T-cells a particular peptide aminoacid sequence derived from a particular protein in a highly specific manner in the polymorphic "groove" of the molecular complex (Rotzschke et al. 1990; Falk et al. 1991; Rammensee et al. 1995, 1999). Each individual carries a set of six different HLA I and six different HLA-II alleles with a defined capacity to present antigens (peptides) to T lymphocytes. HLA class I interacts with the T cell receptor of CD8 positive lymphocytes and HLA class II with the same structure in CD4 positive lymphocytes. In addition, HLA-I molecules also have the ability to interact with Natural Killer (NK) cells, but in this case inhibiting their function (Fig. 1.2). This interaction is regulated by a set of NK receptors that recognize HLA-I molecules: a soubgroup of HLA-B locus products (HLA Bw4 positive alleles) and HLA-Cw molecules as two different entities, i.e. HLA-C1 and HLA-C2 (Moretta et al. 1996; Lanier and Philips 1996; Lanier 2005). The non-classical HLA-E is also interacting with a specific NK cell receptor named CD94/NKG2D (Lopez-Botet and Bellon 1999). NK receptors do not recognize HLA-I allelic differences like T cell receptor do.

The MHC genes and molecules in mice are known as H-2 and are located in chromosome seventeen. The H-2 system was discovered by Peter Gorer in 1935–1936 doing tumour transplantation in different imbread strains of mice (Gorer 1936, 1937). Inbred mice are homozygous and both chromosomes carry the same genes. The commontly used laboratory mice present the H-2 haplotypes H-2^d (BALB/c), H-2^k (CBA/H), H-2^b (C57/BL6), H-2^a (A/Jax), among others. There are two loci for class I: K and D that

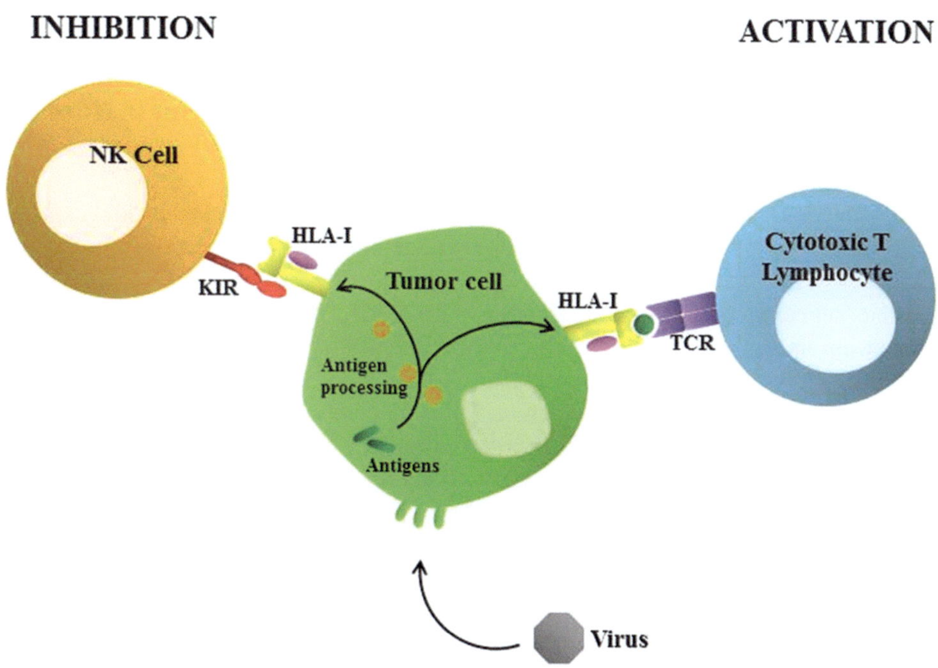

Fig. 1.2 Interaction of HLA class I molecules with T and NK cell receptors. Tumor cells and virus infected cells present tumor antigens to CD8 positive T lymphocytes as nine-aminoacide tumor peptides situated inside the HLA class-I molecule structure. At the same time, HLA-I molecules expressed on the tumor cell surface interact with NK cell receptors inhibiting their function. So, HLA class I molecules can activate T cell function and at the same time inhibit NK cell cytotoxicity

code for two different H-2 class-I molecules. Interestingly, the BALB/c strain (H-2^d) has three loci: K^d, D^d and L^d. George Snell and coworkers in the Jackson laboratories in Bar Harbor (USA) developed the inbred strain of mice and analysed in detail the H-2 system (Snell 1958a, b; Snell et al. 1971). For details about the discovery of H-2 system and the different inbred and recombinant strains of mice see the book edited by Jean Klein: "*Biology of the mouse histocompatibility-2 Complex*" (Klein 1975).

1.3 Antigen Processing and Presentation via HLA Class I/II Molecules

Intracellular antigens derived from viral infections or mutated tumour proteins are presented to T lymphocytes via MHC/HLA class I molecules as nine aminoacid peptides. This important biological process is known as "*Antigen Processing*" (Pamer and Cresswell 1998; Yewdell et al. 2003). MHC/HLA-I molecules are involved mainly in endogenous antigen processing (Townsend and Bodmer 1989). The first event to consider is the proteolitic degradation of the antigen into small fragments capable of forming stable complexes with the corresponding MHC-I molecules. In this enzymatic protein fragmentation, the complex known as proteasome plays an important role. These antigenic peptides are translocated into the Endoplasmic Reticulum (ER) by the transporter associated with antigen processing "TAP1 and TAP2". The HLA class I/β2m complex formation in the ER is carried out with help of chaperons, such as ERp57, calnexin and calreticulin (Harris et al. 1998). Ubiquitinated proteins are degraded by the proteasomes or immune proteasomes into peptides (see Fig. 1.3). Finally, the stable HLA class I/β2m complex is transported via the Golgi apparatus to the cell surface where antigens (peptides) are presented for recognition to CD8+ T cells via the T cell receptor. This biological process allows T lymphocytes to monitor DNA changes/mutations and the elimination of virus infected and transformed cells.

MHC/HLA class II molecules are mostly responsible for the presentation of exogenous antigens to CD4 positive T lymphocytes. They receive peptides generated by the endocytic protein-processing pathway and associate with a protein, i.e. the invariant chain that stops the premature loading of peptides. They both travel to the cytoplasm to interact with endosomes and their cargo of exogenous proteins. They fuse and the exogenous proteins are degraded by proteases. Finally, the peptides derived from exogenous proteins bind the HLA class II groove (Parham 1999). The bacteria previously captured and lysed by the cell via endocytosis are degraded into small fragments of 10 to 12 aminoacids and bind to HLA class II alleles in the cytosol. The exogenous antigens are mostly represented by bacteria and HLA class II antigen presentation is required for CD4 T cells to interact with B cells to produce specific antibodies. It is also accepted that released tumor antigens captured by dendritic cells can be presented by HLA Class II molecules to CD4+ T cells.

1.4 The Expression of HLA-I and II Molecules in Normal Tissues

In order to study HLA class I and II expression in tumor tissues, first it is necessary to study the distribution of HLA class I (A,B,C) and class II (DR,DP,DQ) locus products in different healthy tissues of the body. However, there are few studies that have tried to answer the question: "what human tissues express HLA class I and II molecules"? In 1970 Berah et al reported the first study of HLA in human organs using two alloantisera (Berah et al. 1970). In 1981 Fleming et al used for the first time a monoclonal antibody recognizing a monomorphic determinant of HLA A,B,C molecules and showed that these molecules are not uniformely distributed in all nucleated cells (Fleming et al. 1981). An extensive study was reported by Daar et al in 1984 using the monoclonal antibody PA2.6 (see Table 1.1) (Daar et al. 1984a).

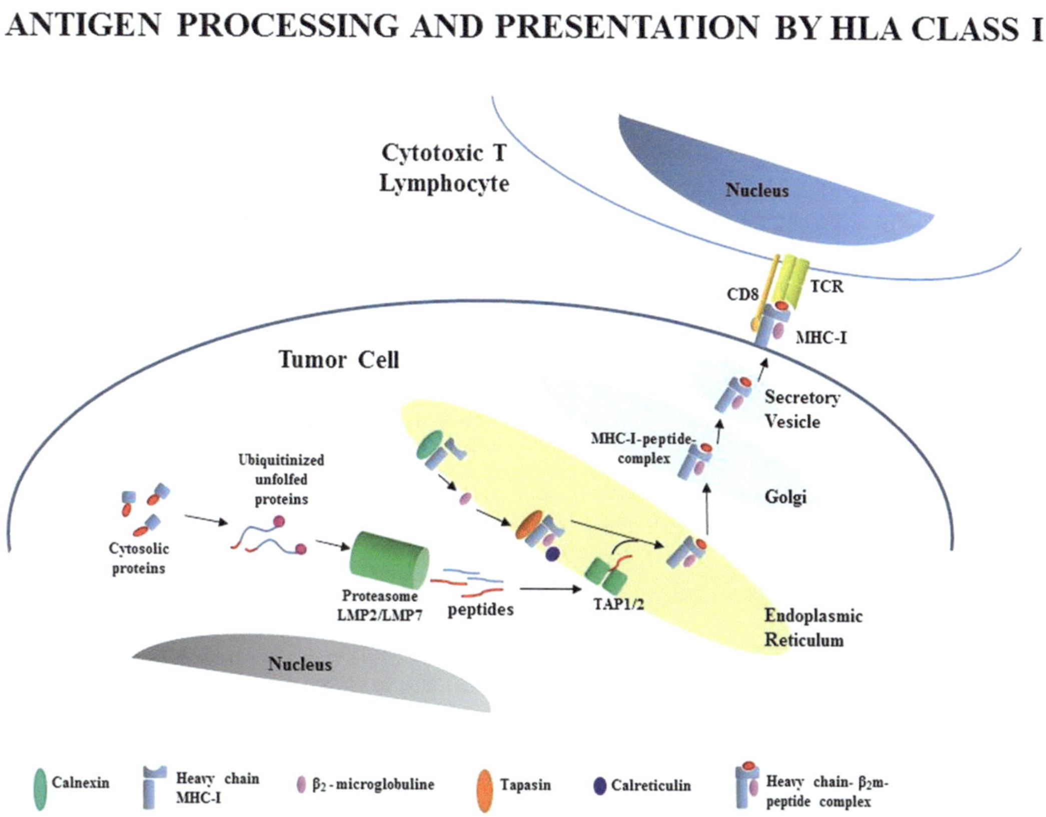

Fig. 1.3 Intracellular Antigen Processing via HLA class I of viral or tumor proteins. Endogenous cellular proteins derived from virus infections or tumor DNA mutations are processed intracellularly and cleaved into peptides. Such peptides are transported into the Endoplasmic Reticulum and bound to HLA class I molecules that are finally exported to the cell surface to interact with CD8 positive T lymphocytes and NK cell receptors

Normal tissues in the gastrointestinal tract, respiratory, cardiovascular and the urogenital systems are HLA class I positive. Hepatocites and skeletal muscles are weakly positive while neurons, the exocrine portion of the pancreas and the cornea endothelium are negative. The antibody PA2.6 used for these studies was later identified as reacting similarly as w6/32 that recognize an epitope on HLA-A,B,C heavy chain/β2 microglobulin complex in the membrane of cells (Brodsky et al. 1979). In 1991, Cordon Cardo also reported the HLA expression in normal tissues when comparing with the expression in different human carcinomas (breast, kidney and bladder) (Cordon-Cardo et al. 1991). This study was important because it confirmed the different patterns of HLA expression in normal and malignant tissues using the previously mentioned w6/32 monoclonal antibody that recognizes a monomorphic framework determinant of HLA heavy chain/β2 microglobulin complex. Normal breast, kidney and bladder epithelia were positive. In our HLA tumor studies we had the opportunity to analyze the HLA-A,B, and C locus-specific transcription in normal tissues such as peripheral blood lymphocytes, colon and laryngeal normal mucosa (Garcia-Ruano et al. 2010). We found clear differences in HLA-A versus B and C locus transcription indicating that this should be further investigated. A detailed analysis of HLA-I ABC locus specific expression in different tissues is not yet available. It is important to emphazise that HLA class-I "cell surface" expression must not be confused with "intracytoplasmic" expression detected with antibodies that measure HLA-ABC free heavy chain inside the cell. In our human tumor studies we always use the HLA class-I expression in the "*tumor stroma*" as a positive internal control. The tumor stroma is composed of different mononuclear cells including T lymphocytes, fibroblasts, and macrophages that are HLA class-I positive.

HLA class II molecules have a more restricted tissue distribution. It is well established that HLA class II molecules (DR, DP, DQ) are expressed in B lymphocytes, macrophages, dendritic cells, or antigen presenting cells. The distribution of HLA class II antigens in normal tissues was also reported by Daar and coworkers (Daar et al. 1984b). Some ephitelia that line the outer surfaces of organs are also HLA class II positive (see Table 1.1). We are still lacking adetailed analysis of HLA class II, including the DR, DQ and DP molecule expression in different human tissues.

References

Alcami A, Koszinowski UH (2000) Viral mechanisms of immune evasion. Immunol Today 21(9):447–455

Allison JP, McIntyre BW, Bloch D (1982) Tumor specific antigen of murine T-lymphoma defined with monoclonal antibody. J Immunol 129(5):2293–2300

Allison JP, Hurwitz AA, Leach D (1995) Manipulation of costimulatory signals to enhance anti-tumor T-cell responses. Curr Opin Immunol 7(5):682–686

Amos B (1986) Recollections of Dr Peter Gorer. Immunogenetics 24(6):341–344

Andersen R, Donia M, Ellebaek E, Holz Borch T, Kongsted P, Iversen TZ, Rosenkrantz Hölmich L, Westergren Hendel H, Met O, Hald AM, thor Straten P, Svane IM (2016) Long-lasting complete responses in patients with metastatic melanoma after adoptive cell therapy with tumor-infiltrating lymphocytes and an attenuated IL-2 regimen. Clin Cancer Res 22(15):3734–3745

Aptsiauri N, Cabrera T, Pawelec G, Gouttefangeas C, Derhovanessian E, Garrido F, Garcia-Lora A (2007a) International conference: progress in vaccination against cancer 2006 (PIVAC 6) Granada, Spain. Cancer Immunol Immunother 56:1311–1322

Aptsiauri N, Cabrera T, Garcia-Lora A, Lopez-Nevot MA, Ruiz-Cabello F, Garrido F (2007b) MHC class I antigens and immune surveillance in transformed cells. Int Rev Cytol 256:139–189

Aptsiauri N, Cabrera T, Garcia-Lora A, Ruiz-Cabello F, Garrido F (2008) HLA class I expression, tumour escape and cancer progression. Curr Cancer Ther Rev 5:105–110

Aptsiauri N, Cabrera T, Garcia-Lora A, Garrido F (2012) Cancer immune escape: implications for immunotherapy, Granada, Spain, October 3–5, 2011. Cancer Immunol Immunother 61(5):739–745

Aptsiauri N, Ruiz-Cabello F, Garrido F (2018) The transition from HLA-I positive to HLA-I negative primary tumors: the road to escape from T cell responses. Curr Opin Immunol 51:123–132

Baldwin RW (1955) Immunity to methylcholanthrene-induced tumors in inbred rats following atrophy and regression of implanted tumors. Br J Cancer 9:652–657

Basombrio MA (1970) Search for common antigenicities among twenty-five sarcomas induced by methylcholanthrene. Cancer Res 30:2458–2462

Berah M, Hors J, Dausset J (1970) A study of HLA antigens in human organs. Transplantation 9:185

Boesen M, Svane IM, Engel AM, Rygaard J, Thomsen AR, Werdelin O (2000) CD8+ T cells are crucial for the ability of congenic normal mice to reject highly immunogenic sarcomas induced in nude mice with 3-methylcholantrene. Clin Exp Immunol 121:210–215

Bjorkman PJ, Saper MA, Samraoui B, Bennett WS, Strominger JL, Wiley DC (1987) Structure of the human class I histocompatibility antigen, HLA-A2. Nature 329(6139):506–512

Bodmer WF, Browning MJ, Krausa P, Rowan A, Bicknell DC, Bodmer JG (1993) Tumour escape from immune response by variation in HLA expression and other mechanisms. Ann NY Acad Sci 690:422–449

Boon T (1983) Antigenic tumor cell variants obtained with mutagens. Adv Cancer Res 39:121–151

Boon T, Cerottini JC, Van den Eynde B, van der Bruggen P, Van Pel A (1994) Tumor antigens recognized by T lymphocytes. Annu Rev Immunol 12:337–365

Boon T, van der Bruggen P (1996) Human tumor antigens recognized by T lymphocytes. J Exp Med 183:725–729

Boon T, Coulie P, Van Den Eynde BJ, Van Der Bruggen P (2006) Human T cell responses against melanoma. Annu Rev Immunol 24:175–208

Brodsky F, Parham P, Barnstable C, Crumpton M, Bodmer WF (1979) Monoclonal antibodies for analysis of the HLA system. Immunol Rev 47:3–61

Buferne M, Chasson L, Grange M, Mas A, Arnoux F, Bertuzzi M, Naquet P, Leserman L, Schmitt-Verhulst AM (2015) Auphan-Anezin N (2015) IFN-g producing CD8+ cells modified to resist major immune checkpoints induce regression of MHC class I-deficient melanomas. Oncoimmunology 4:e974759

Burnet FM (1957) Cancer: a biological approach. Brit Med J I:779–786

Burnet FM (1970) The concept of immunological surveillance. Prog Exp Tumor Res 13:1–27

Burnet FM (1971) Immunological surveillance in neoplasia. Transplant Rev 7:3–25

Butcher G (1986) Editorial. J Immunogenet 13(2/3)

Cabrera T, Ruiz-Cabello F, Garrido F (1995) Biological implications of HLA-DR expression in tumours. Scand J Immunol 41:398–406

Cabrera T, Lopez-Nevot MA, Gaforio JJ, Ruiz-Cabello F, Garrido F (2003) Analysis of HLA expression in human tumor tissues. Cancer Immunol Immunother 52(1):1–9

Chomez P, De Backer O, Bertrand M, De Plaen E, Boon T, Lucas S (2001) An overview of the MAGE gene family with the identification of all human members of the family. Cancer Res 61:5544–5551

Chowell D, Morris L, Grigg C, Weber J, Samstein R, Makarov V, Kuo F, Kendall S, Requena D, Riaz N, Greenbaum B, Carroll J, Garon E, Hyman D, Zehir A, Solit D, Berger M, Zhou R, Rizvi N, Chan T (2017) Patient HLA class I genotype influences cancer response to checkpoint blockade immunotherapy. Science. https://doi.org/10.1126/science.aao4572

Cordon-Cardo C, Fuks Z, Drobnjak M, Moreno C, Eisenbach L, Feldman M (1991) Expression of HLA-A,B,C antigens on primary and metastatic tumor cell populations of human carcinomas. Cancer Res 51:6372–6380

Csiba A, Whitwell HL, Moore M (1984) Distribution of histocompatibility and leukocyte differentiation antigens in normal human colon and in benign and malignant colonic neoplasms. Br J Cancer 50:699–709

Daar AS, Fuggle SV, Fabre JV, Ting A, Morris PJ (1984a) The detailed distribution of HLA-A,B,C antigens in normal human organs. Transplantation 38(3):287–292

Daar AS, Fuggle SV, Fabre JV, Ting A, Morris PJ (1984b) The detailed distribution of MHC class II antigens in normal human organs. Transplantation 38(3):293–298

Dausset J (1954) Leucoagglutinins IV.- Leucoagglutinins and blood transfusions. Vox Sang 4:190–194

Dausset J (1958) Iso-leuco-anticorps. Acta Haematologica (Basel). 20:156–160

David CS (1987) H-2 antigens: genes, molecules, function, Nato ASI series, Series A: life sciences, 144. Plenum Press, New York/London

Dunn GP, Bruce AT, Ikeda H, Old LJ, Schreiber RD (2002) Cancer immunoediting: from immunosurveillance to tumor escape. Nat Immunol 11:991–998

Dunn GP, Old LJ, Schreiber RD (2004) The three Es of cancer immunoediting. Annu Rev Immunol 22:329–360

Falk K, Rotzschke O, Stevanovic S, Jung G, Rammensee HG (1991) Allele-specific motifs revealed by sequencing of self-peptides eluted from MHC molecules. Nature 351:290–296

Fleming KA, McMichael A, Morton JA, Woods J, McGee JO (1981) Distribution of HLA class I antigens in normal human tissue and in mamary cancer. J Clin Pathol 34:779–785

Festenstein H, Schmidt W (1981) Variation in MHC antigen profiles of tumour cells and its biological effects. Immunol Rev 60:85

Festenstein H, Garrido F (1986) MHC antigens and malignancy. Nature 322:502–523

Festenstein H (1987) The biological consequences of altered MHC expression on tumours. Br Med Bull 43:217–227

Foley EJ (1953) Antigenic properties of methylcholanthrene induced tumors in mice of the strain of origin. Cancer Res 13:835–837

Garcia-Ruano AB, Méndez R, Romero JM, Cabrera T, Ruiz-Cabello F, Garrido F (2010) Analysis of HLA-ABC locus-specific transcription in normal tissues. Immunogenetics 62(11–12):711–719

Garrido F, Festenstein H, Schirrmacher V (1976) Further evidence for derepression of H-2 and Ia-like specificities of foreign haplotypes in mouse tumour cell lines. Nature 261:705–707

Garrido F, Schirrmacher V, Festenstein H (1977) Studies on H-2 specificities on mouse tumour cells by a new microradioassay. J Immunogenet 4:15–27

Garrido F, Perez M, Torres MD (1979) Absence of four H-2^d antigenic specificites in an H-2^d sarcoma. J Immunogenet 6(2):83–86

Garrido F (1991) MHC molecules in normal and neoplastic cells. Introduction. Int J Cancer, Supplement 6, 1

Garrido F, Klein E (1991) MHC antigen expression I. Human tumors. Seminars in cancer biology, vol 2, no 1. Klein E, Garrido F, eds. Saunders Scientific Publications, pp 1–2

Garrido F, Cabrera T, Concha A, Glew S, Ruiz-Cabello F, Stern P (1993) Natural history of HLA antigens during tumour development. Immunol Today 14(10):491–499

Garrido F, Cabrera T, Lopez-Nevot MA, Ruiz-Cabello F (1995) HLA class I antigens in human tumors. Adv Cancer Res 67:155–195

Garrido F (1996) Editorial, HLA and cancer. Tissue Antigens 47(5):361–363

Garrido F, Ruiz-Cabello F, Cabrera T, Perez-Villar JJ, Lopez-Botet M, Duggan-Keen M, Stern P (1997) Altered HLA-I phenotypes in human tumors: implication for immunesurveillance. Immunol Today 18(2):89–95

Garrido F, Algarra I (2001) MHC antigens and tumor escape from immune surveillance. Adv Cancer Res 83:117–158

Garrido F, Aptsiauri N, Doorduijn E, Garcia-Lora A, van Hall T (2016) The urgent need to recover MHC class I in cancers for effective immunotherapy. Curr Opin Immunol 39:44–51

Gorer PA (1936) The detection of antigenic diferences in mouse erythrocytes by the employment of immune sera. Br J Exp Pathol 17:42–55

Gorer PA (1937) The genetic and antigenic basis of tumor transplantation. J Pathol Bacteriol 44:691–697

Gorer PA, Mikulska ZB (1954) The antibody response to tumor inoculation. Improved methods of antibody detection. Cancer Res 14:651–655

Gorer PA, O'Gorman P (1956) The cytotoxic activity of isoantibodies in mice. Transplant Bull 3:142–143

Grasso C, Giannakis M, Wells DK, Hamada T, Mu J, Quist M, Nowak JA, Nishihara R, Qian ZR, Inamura K et al (2018) Genetic mechanisms of immune evasion in colorectal cancer. Cancer Discov. https://doi.org/10.1158/2159-8290.CD-17-1327

Gross L (1943) Intradermal immunization of C3H mice against a sarcoma that originated in an animal of the same line. Cancer Res 3:326–333

Hansen J (2006) Immunobiology of the human MHC. In: Proceedings of the 13th international histocompatibil-

ity workshop and conference, Victoria BC 2002 (Ed. John Hansen, 2006, IHWC Press)
Harris MR, Yu Y, Kindle CS, Hansen TH, Solheim JC (1998) Calreticulin and calnexin interact with different protein and glycan determinants during the assembly of MHC class I. J Immunol. 160:5404–5409
Kärre K, Ljunggren HJ, Piontek G, Kiessling (1986) Selective rejection of H-2 deficient lymphoma variants suggests alternative immune defence strategy. Nature 319:675–678
Kärre K (1997) How to recognize a foreign submarine. Immunol Rev 155:5–9
Klein G, Sjogren HO, Klein E, Hellstrom KE (1960) Demonstration of resistance against methylcholanthrene induced sarcomas in the primary autochtonous host. Cancer Res 20:1561–1157
Klein J (1975) Biology of the mouse histocompatibility-2 complex. Principles of immunogenetics applied to a single system. Springer, New York
Klein J (1986) Seeds of time: fifty years ago Peter Gorer discovered the H-2 complex. Immunogenetics 24(6):331–338
Klein J, Sato A (2000a) The HLA system: first of two parts. N Engl J Med 7:702–709
Klein J, Sato A (2000b) The HLA system: second of two parts. N Engl J Med 14:782–786
Kiessling R, Klein E, Wigzell H (1975) "Natural Killer" cells in the mouse.I.- Cytotoxic cells with specificity for mouse Moloney leukemia cells. Specificity and distribution according to genotype. Eur J Immunol 5(2):112–117
Kiessling R, Wigzell H (1979) An analysis of the murine NK cell as to structure, function and biological relevance. Immunol Rev 44:165
Kvistborg P, Philips D, Kelderman S, Hageman L, Ottensmeier C, Joseph-Pietras D, Welters M, van de Burg S, Kapiteijn E, Michielin O et al (2014) Anti CTL-4 therapy broadens the melanoma-reactive CD8+ T cell response. Sci Transl Med 6:1–9
Lampen M, van Hall T (2011) Strategies to counteract MHC-I defects in tumors. Curr Opin Immunol 23:293–298
Lanier LL, Philips JH (1996) Inhibitory MHC class I receptors on NK cells and T cells. Immunol Today 17:86–91
Lanier LL (2005) NK cell recognition. Annu Rev Immunol 23:225–274
Leach D, Krummel MF, Allison JP (1996) Enhancement of antitumor immunity by CTLA-4 blockade. Science 271(5256):1734–11736
Ljunggren HG, Kärre K (1986) Experimental strategies and interpretations in the analysis of changes in MHC gene expression during tumour progression: opposing influences of T cell and natural killer cell mediated resistance? J Immunogenet 13(2/3):141–151
Ljunggren HG, Kärre K (1990) In search of the 'missing self': MHC molecules and NK cell recognition. Immunol Today 11(7):237–244
Lopez-Botet M, Bellon T (1999) Natural killer cell activation and inhibition by receptors for MHC class I. Curr Opin Immunol 11:301–307
Lopez-Nevot MA, Garcia E, Pareja E, Bonal J, Martin F, Ruiz-Cabello F, Serrano S, Garrido F (1986) Differential expression of HLA class I and II antigens in primary and metastatic melanomas. J Immunogenet 13:219–227
Lopez-Nevot MA, Esteban F, Ferron A, Gutierrez J, Oliva MR, Romero C, Huelin C, Ruiz-Cabello F, Garrido F (1989) HLA class I gene expression on human primary tumours and autologous metastases: demonstration of selective losses of HLA antigens on colorectal, gastric and laryngeal carcinomas. Br J Cancer 59:221–226
McGranahan N, Rosenthal R, Hiley CT, Rowan AJ, Watkins TBK, Wilson GA, Birkbak NJ, Veeriah S, Van Loo P, Herrero J, Swanton C (2017) TRACERx consortium, allele-specific HLA loss and immune escape in lung cancer evolution. Cell 171:1259–1271.e11. https://doi.org/10.1016/j.cell.2017.10.001Medline
Marchand M, Van baren N, Weynan P, Brichard V, Dreno B, Tessier MH, Rankin E, Parmiani G, Arienti F, Humblet Y et al (1999) Tumour regression observed in patients with metastatic melanoma treated with an antigenic peptide encoded by gene MAGE-3 and presented by HLA-A1. Int J Cancer 80:219–230
Marincola FM, Jafee EM, Hicklin DJ, Ferrone (2000) Escape of human solid tumors from T-cell recognition: molecular mechanisms and functional significance. Adv Immunol 74:181–273
Milstein C (1987) Introductory remarks. Leucocyte Typing III. White Cell differentiation Antigens. McMichael AJ (ed). Oxford University Press, Oxford
Moore M, Ghosh AK, Johnston D, Street AJ (1986) Expression of MHC class II products on human colorectal cancer. An immunohistological and flow cytometric study. J Immunogenet 13:201–209
Morales A, Eidinger D, Bruce AW (1976) Intracavitary Bacillus Calmette Guerin in the treatment of superficial bladder tumors. J Urol 116(2):180–183
Moretta A, Bottino C, Vitale M, Pende D, Biassoni R, Mingari MC, Moretta L (1996) Receptors for HLA class I molecules in human natural killer cells. Annu Rev Immunol 14:619–648
Nakazato H, Koike A, Saji S, Ogawa N, Sakamoto J (1994) Efficacy of immunochemotherapy as adjuvant treatment after curative resection of gastric cancer. Lancet 143:1122–1124
Natali PG, Cavaliere R, Bigotti A, Nicotra MR, Russo C, Giacomini P, Ferrone S (1983) Antigenic heterogeneity of surgically removed primary and autologous metastatic human melanoma lesions. J Immunol 130(3):1462–1466
Natali PG, Bigotti A, Nicotra MR, Viora M, Manfredi D, Ferrone S (1984) Distribution of human class I (HLA-A,B,C) histocompatibility antigens in normal and malignant tissues of nonlymphoid origin. Cancer Res 44:4679–4687
Natali PG, Nicotra MR, Bigotti A, Venturo I, Marcenaro L, Giacomini P, Russo C (1989) Selective changes

in expression of HLA class I polymorphic determinants in human solid tumors. Proc Natl Acad Sci USA 86(17):6719–6723

Nestle FO, Alijagic S, Gilliet M, Sun Y, Grabbe S, Dummer R, Burg G, Shadendorf D (1998) Vaccination of melanoma patients with peptide of tumour lysate-pulsed dendritic cells. Nature Medicine 4:328–332

Nio Y, Shiraishi T, Tsubono M, Morimoto H, Tseng C, Imai S, Tobe T (1991) In vitro immunomodulating effect of protein-bound polysaccharide K on peripheral blood, regional nodes and spleen lymphocytes in patients with gastric cancer. Cancer Immunol Immunother 32:335–341

Pamer E, Cressswell P (1998) Mechanism of MHC class I-restricted antigen processing. Annu Rev Immunol 16:323–358

Parham P (1999) Pathways of antigen processing and presentation, Immunological Reviews, Vol 172. Munksgaard, Copenhagen

Prehn RT, Main JM (1957) Immunity to methylcholanthrene induced sarcomas. J Natl Cancer Inst 18:769–778

Rammensee HG, Friede T, Stevanovich S (1995) MHC ligands and peptide motifs: First listing. Immunogenetics 41:178–228

Rammensee H, Bachmann J, Emmerich NP, Bachor OA, Stevanovic S (1999) SYFPEITHI: database for MHC ligands and peptide motifs. Immunogenetics 50:213–219

Romero P, Coulie P (2014) Adaptive T cell immunity and tumor antigen recognition. In: Rees R (ed) Tumor immunology and immunotherapy. Oxford University Press, Oxford, pp 1–14

Rosenberg SA, Lotze MT, Muul, Chang AE, Avis FP, Leitman S, Linehan WM, Robertson CN, Lee RE, Rubin TJ et al (1987) A progress report on the treatment of 157 patients with advance cancer using lymphokine-activated killer cells and interleukin-2 or high-dose interleukin-2 alone. N Engl J Med 316(15):889–897

Rosenberg SA, Yang JC, Sherry RM, Kammula US, Hughes MS, Phan GQ, Citrin DE, Restifo NP, Robbins PF, Wunderlich JR, Morton KE, Laurencot CM, Steinberg SM, White DE, Dudley ME (2011) Durable complete responses in heavily pretreated patients with metastatic melanoma using T-cell transfer immunotherapy. Clin Cancer Res 17:4550–4557

Rotzschke O, Flak K, Deres K, Schild H, Norda M, Metzger J, Jung G, Ramansee HG (1990) Isolation and analysis of naturally processed viral peptides as recognized by cytotoxic T cells. Nature 15(348):252–254

Ruiter DJ, Bhan AK, Harrist TJ, Sober AJ, Mihm MC (1982) Major histocompatibility antigens and mononuclear inflammatory infiltrate in benign novomelanocytic proliferations and malignant melanoma. J Immunol 129:2808–2815

Ruiter DJ, Bergman W, Welvaart K, Scheffer E, van Vloten WA, Russo C, Ferrone S (1984) Immunohistochemical analysis of malignant melanomas and nevocellular nevi with monoclonal antibodies to distinct monomorphic determinants of HLA antigens. Cancer Res 14:3930–3936

Ruiter DJ, Brocker E, Ferrone S (1986) Expression and susceptibility to modulation by interferons of HLA class I and II antigens on melanoma cells. Immunohistochemical analysis and clinical relevance. J Immunogenet 13:229–234

Ruiz-Cabello F, Garrido F (2002) Tumor evasion of the immune system. In: Parmiani, Lotze (eds) Tumor immunology: molecular defined antigens and clinical applications. Taylor and Francis, Routledge, pp 177–203

Schmidt W, Atfield G, Festenstein H (1979) Loss of H-2K^k gene products from several AKR spontaneous leukemias. Immunogenetics 8:311

Schmidt W, Festenstein H (1982) Resistance to cell-mediated cytotoxicity is corrclated with reduction of H-2K gene products in AKR leukemia. Immunogenetics 16:257–264

Schrier P, Bernars R, Vaessen RTMJ, Houweling A, van der Erb AJ (1983) Expression of class I major histocompatibility antigens swiched off by highly oncogenic adenovirus 12 in transformed rat cells. Nature 305:771–775

Snell G (1958a) Histocompatibility genes of the mouse. I. Demonstration of weak histocompatibility differences by immunization and controlled tumour dosage. J Nat Cancer Inst 20:787–824

Snell G (1958b) Histocompatibility genes of the mouse II. Production and analysis of isogenic resistant lines. J Natl Cancer Inst 21:843–877

Snell G, Cherry M, Demant P (1971) Evidence that H-2 private specificities can be arrange in two mutually exclusive systems possibly homologous with two subsystems of HL-A. Transplant Proc 3:183–186

Snell GD (1986) Some recollections of Peter Gorer and his work on this fiftieth anniversary of his discovery of H-2. Immunogenetics 24(6):339–340

Smith MEF, Marsh SGE, Bodmer JG, Gelsthorpe K, Bodmer WF (1989) Loss of HLA-A,B,C allele products and lymphocyte function-associated antigen 3 in colorectal neoplasia. Proc Natl Acad Sci USA 86:5557–5561

Stern LJ, Wiley DC (1994) Antigenic peptide binding by class I and class II histocompatibility proteins. Structure 2:245–251

Sucker A, Zhao F, Pieper N, Heeke C, Maltaner R, Stadtler N, Real B, Bielefeld N, Howe S, Weide B, Gutzmer R, Utikal J, Loquai C, Gogas H, Klein-Hitpass L, Zeschnigk M, Westendorf A, Trilling M, Horn S, Schilling B, Schadendorf D, Griewank K, Paschen A (2017) Adquired IFNγ resistance impairs anti-tumor immunity and gives rise to T-cell-resistance melanoma lesions. Nat Commun 8:15440. https://doi.org/10.1038/ncomms15440

Svane IM, Boesen M, Engel AM (1999) The role of cytotoxic T lymphocytes in prevention and immune surveillance of tumor. Lessons from normal and immunedeficient mice. Med Oncol 16(4):223–238

Thor Straten P, Garrido F (2016) Targetless T cells in cancer immunotherapy. J Immunother Cancer 4:23–26
Thomas L (1959) Cellular and humoral aspects of hypersensitivity. Lawrence HS (ed). Hoeber-Harper, New York
Townsend A, Rothbard J, Gotch FM, Bahadur G, Wrath D, McMichael AJ (1986) The epitopes of influenza nucleoprotein recognized by cytotoxic T lymphocytes can be defined with short synthetic peptides. Cell 44:959–968
Townsend A, Bodmer H (1989) Antigen recognition by class-I restricted T lymphocytes. Annu Rev Immunol 7:601–624
Van der Bruggen P, Traversary C, Chomez P, Lurquin C, De Plaen E, Van den Eynde B, Knuth A, Boon T (1991) A gene encoding an antigen recognized by cytolitic T lymphocytes on a human melanoma. Science 254:1643–1647
Van Rood JJ. (1962) Leucocyte Grouping: a method and its application. Doctoral thesis, Leiden University
Villunger A, Strasser A (1999) The great escape: Is immune evasion required for tumor progression? Nat Med 5:874–875
Yewdell JW, Reits E, Neefjes J (2003) Making sense of mass destruction: quantitating MHC class I antigen presentation. Nat Rev Immunol 3:952–961
Zinkernagel RM, Doherty PC (1974) Restriction of in vitro T cell-mediated cytotoxicity in lymphocytic choriomeningitis within a syngeneic or semiallogeneic system. Nature 248(5450):701–702
Zinkernagel RM, Doherty PC (1979) MHC-restricted cytotoxic T cells: studies on the biological role of polymorphic major transplantation antigens determining T-cell-restricted specificity, function and responsiveness. Adv Immunol 27:51–177
Zinkernagel RM (1996) Cellular immune recognition and the biological role of major transplantation antigens. Nobel lecture, December 8
Zinkernagel, Doherty (1997) The discovery of MHC restriction. Immunol Today 18:14–17

MHC/HLA Class I Loss in Cancer Cells

2

Abstract

In this chapter I describe Tumour Immune Escape mechanisms associated with MHC/HLA class I loss in human and experimental tumours. Different altered HLA class-I phenotypes can be observed that are produced by different molecular mechanisms. Experimental and histological evidences are summarized indicating that at the early stages of tumour development there is an enormous variety of tumour clones with different MHC class I expression patterns. This phase is followed by a strong T cell mediated immune-selection of MHC/HLA class-I negative tumour cells in the primary tumour lesion. This transition period results in a formation of a tumour composed only of HLA-class I negative cells. An updated description of this process observed in a large variety of human tumors is included. In the second section I focus on MHC/HLA class I alterations observed in mouse and human metastases, and describe the generation of different tumor cell clones with altered MHC class I phenotypes, which could be similar or different from the original tumor clone. The biological and immunological relevance of these observations is discussed. Finally, the interesting phenomenon of metastatic dormancy is analyzed in association with a particular MHC class I negative tumor phenotype.

Keywords

Primary tumors · T lymphocytes · NK cells · HLA-I in tissues · HLA-I loss in different tumors · Immunohistochemistry · Tumor HLA-I phenotypes · Tumor rejection · Tumor escape · Tumor dormancy · HLA-I in metastasis · Tumor infiltrating lymphocytes · Tumor tissue architecture

There is strong evidence that cancer cells grow and metastazise despite an active immune response by the tumor bearing host. T lymphocytes can recognize processed tumor antigens as small peptides presented by HLA-I molecules (Romero and Coulie 2014; Boesen et al. 2000). This recognition and activation ends with the destruction of the solid nascent tumor. The concept of immune surveillance was suggested many years ago by Erlich (1909), and later by Burnet (1957, 1970) and Thomas (1959). Today there is evidence indicating that T lymphocytes are responsible for this surveillance that ends with the recognition and destruction of the aberrant tumor cells (Boon et al. 1994) and cells infected by highly oncogenic viruses (Bernards et al. 1983). The question which immediately comes to mind is: why do tumors arise and develop? Why does immune surveillance fail? Tumour escape strategies are the most likely cause of the failure of T-cell mediated immune surveillance of cancer.

F. Garrido, *MHC Class-I Loss and Cancer Immune Escape*, Advances in Experimental Medicine and Biology 1151, https://doi.org/10.1007/978-3-030-17864-2_2

The failure of immune surveillance against solid tumors was named "immunological ignorance" (Ochsenbein et al. 1999). HLA class I loss or downregulation is undoubtedly playing a leading role in this process (Natali et al. 1984; Garrido 1987; Ruiz-Cabello et al. 1987; Lopez-Nevot et al. 1987; Garrido and Ruiz-Cabello 1991; Cabrera et al. 1991; Algarra et al. 1997; Marincola et al. 2000; Ruiz-Cabello and Garrido 2002; Campoli and Ferrone 2008). In addition, we have observed that MHC class I molecules can act as tumor suppressor genes regulating the cell cycle gene expression, invasion and intrinsic tumorigenicity of tumor cells (Garrido et al. 2012). It is important to bear in mind that HLA class I total loss or selective dowregulation is not the only mechanism associated with tumor immune escape. Indeed, different tumor escape strategies have been described in solid tumors or tumor cell lines such as: (a) loss of tumor antigen expression (Jager et al. 1996) (b) resistance of tumor cells to γ or α interferon stimulation due to mutations of different genes responsible for the IFN signal transduction pathways (Dunn et al. 2005; Rodriguez et al. 2007a, b), (c) upregulation of inhibitors of apoptosis in tumour cells (Catlett-Falcone et al. 1999; Hinz et al. 2000) or promotion of apoptosis in anti-tumor T cells (Dong et al. 2002), (d) generation of immune suppressive factors in the tumor microenviroment and accumulation of regulatory T cells (Terabe and Berzofsky 2004; Sakaguchi et al. 2001), (e) lack of expression of co-estimulatory molecules that lead to failure on the recognition and destruction of tumor cells (Schultze and Nadler 2003) and (f) release of immunosupresive cytokines (Aruga et al. 1997). However, the frequency and clinical relevance of such escape mechanisms in different human tumors is not known.

The first part of this chapter describes the early stages of MHC/HLA-I losses that take place in the "primary tumor niche", including important structural and functional changes in the tumor microenviroment associated with the tumor escape phenotype. We will discuss the transition from HLA-I positive to HLA-I negative tumors, as well as the HLA-I altered phenotypes and the HLA-I expression patterns in different tumor tissues. In the second part, I will describe the changes occuring in H-2 class I expression in the "spontaneous metastasis" obtained in the GR9 fibrosarcoma mouse model that we have extensively analyzed for many years in my laboratory in Granada. I will include also in this chapter the HLA analysis of "human metastasis" obtained from different anatomical locations (subcutaneous, lymph nodes, liver…) provided by different clinical departments in my hospital or in cooperation with different European Oncology centers. Finally, I will also focus on discussing the state of "metastatic dormancy" that has been described in mouse experimental models and in humans. Figure 2.1 summarizes three stages of the tumor development identified in mouse and human tumors: rejection, escape and dormancy associated with HLA class I expression or loss (Garrido et al. 2016a).

2.1 MHC/HLA Class I Loss in Primary Tumors

Tumors derive from MHC/HLA class I positive epithelia and remain positive at early stages of tumor development. Later, MHC/HLA-I loss variants appear in primary tumor lesions with tumor clones expressing high, intermediate and low MHC/HLA-I class I expression (Ruiz-Cabello et al. 1991b). This "explosion of diversity" can be detected by different techniques, including immunohistology, and also by flow cytometry of tumor cells isolated from fresh tumors and adapted to tissue culture (Koopman et al. 2000; Garrido et al. 2016b). Anti-tumor immune response mediated by T lymphocytes attacks and destroys tumor cells expressing MHC/HLA-I molecules that present the specific tumor antigen and leaves unharmed MHC/HLA-I negative tumor cells. At the end of this selection process the tumor is composed only of MHC/HLA-I negative cells (see Fig. 2.1). HLA class I loss is a frequent finding in primary tumors and there are indications that might be, indeed, a prerequisite for tumors to develop (Villunger and Strasser 1999). This phenomenon has important implications in

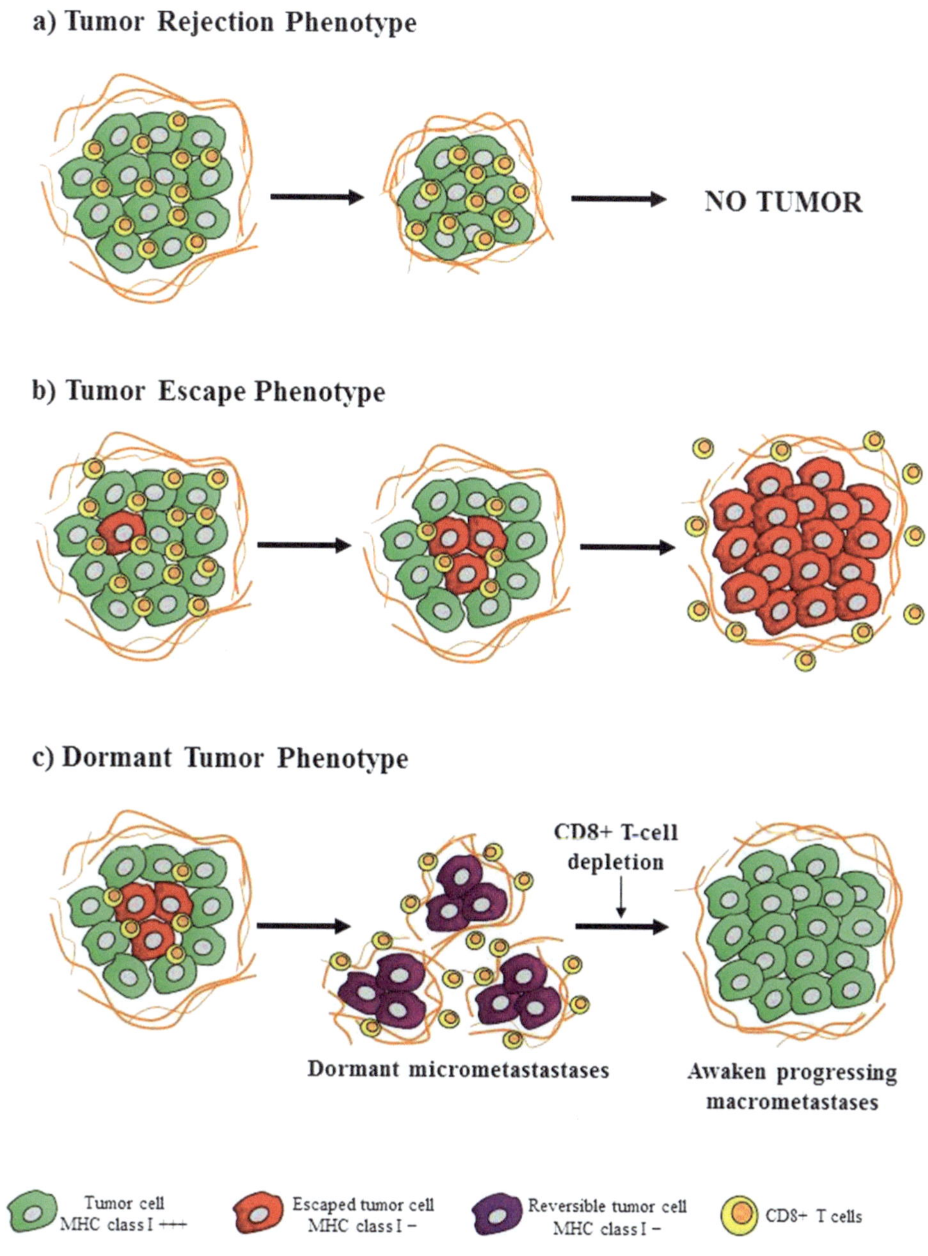

Fig. 2.1 Patterns of HLA-I expression associated with tumor rejection, escape and dormancy. Tumor rejection is associated with antigen presentation ability, high levels of H-2/HLA class I expression and lymphocyte infiltration within the tumour nest (**a**). Tumor escape is linked to the absence or low levels of MHC class I molecules at the tumor cell surface and lymphocytes located in the stroma surrounding the tumor (**b**). Tumor dormancy in metastatic colonies occurs in MHC class-I negative tumor cells that maintain the capability to re-express class I molecules (**c**). (Figure reprinted by permission from Elsevier: Garrido et al. 2016a)

cancer immunotherapy due to the ability of some tumors to recover the expression of the missing HLA-I especificities (Garrido et al. 2010a).

2.1.1 H-2/HLA-I Heterogeneity

MHC tumor heterogeneity is clearly observed in newly induced mouse tumors. In the middle of the

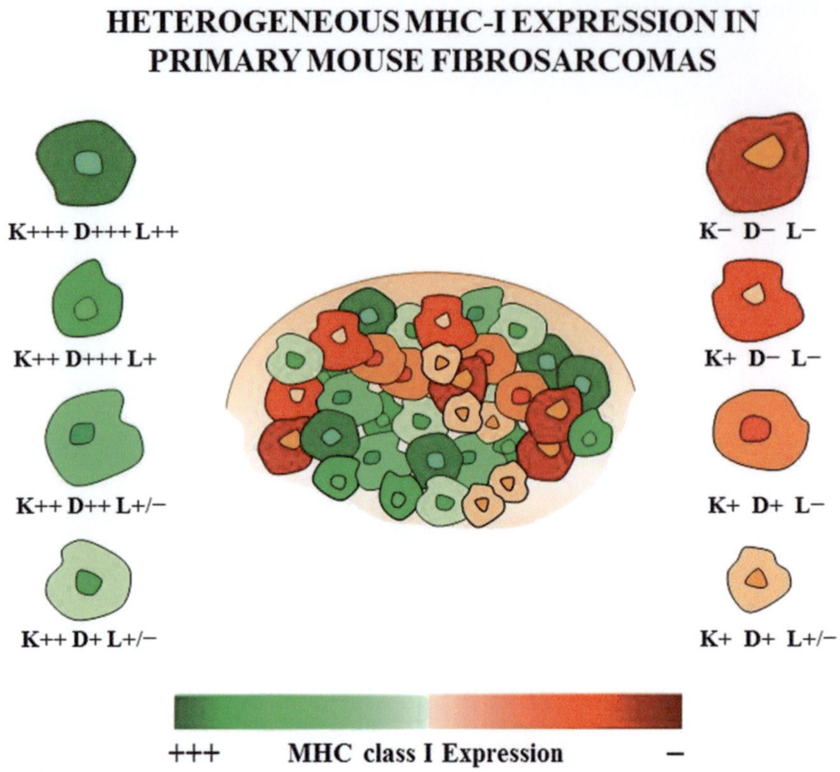

Fig. 2.2 H-2 class I expression in different clones from the GR9 mouse fibrosarcoma originated in a BALB/c mouse. The primary tumor was adapted to tissue culture without any passage "in vivo" to avoid changes in its composition. The tumor cells were cloned and typed for H-2 class-I expression. An enormous variety of clones were identified expressing different amount of H-2 K,D,L molecules i.e. negative, weakly positive, and strongly positive. Similar results were obtained when testing others methylcholantre induced sarcomas. (For details see Garrido et al. 1986a, Algarra et al. 1991, and Garrido et al. 2016b)

80s we produced a large number of methylcholantrene induced sarcomas in different strain of inbread mice, in particular in BALB/c mice. We decided to adapt the solid tumor mass of about 0.5–1 cm in diameter to tissue culture without any passage in syngeneic mice. The idea was to avoid changes in its composition caused by various mechanisms of immunoselection of the host. When these tumors were cloned and typed for H-2 expression using flow cytometry we observed a common pattern i.e. a presence of multiple clones with different cell surface expression of MHC-I antigens (Garrido et al. 1977, 1979, 1986a, b; Algarra et al. 1991). There were clones expressing high, intermediate and low/negative levels of K, D and L molecules (see Fig. 2.2). Hypermethylation of the DNA was found to be associated with the low/negative H-2 class I expressing clones and low level of MHC class I gene transcription (Bonal et al. 1986). This "explosion of diversity" of MHC expression present in different tumor clones is generated in a short period of time. It looks like a "biological big-bang" (Garrido et al. 2016b; Aptsiauri et al. 2008). This variety of MHC expression in tumor clones contrasts with the homogeneous tumor cell lines used in laboratory work that might suggest that tumors are composed by a single clone and that there is no "diversity". The question that can arise is why the long term established tumor cell lines are MHC class I positive? A possibility is that MHC class I positive tumor cell lines can be more easily adapted to tissue culture than MHC class I negative ones. A second one is that the cell surface analysis of HLA is not accurately analyzed, since it requires the study of the six different alleles. A third possibility is that MHC class negative tumor cells are not detected in an heterogenous tumor population composed of positive and negative cells as we observed in our GR9 mouse fibrosarcoma (Garrido et al. 1986a, b, 2016b).

I favour the idea that the primary tumor is composed of multiple clones with multiple different cell markers and different biological properties. We have focused on MHC cell surface expression, but probably any other marker would also be differentially expressed. An important question is: are we dealing with different individual tumors with different immunological properties? The answer is "no", because the tumor clones obtained can cross-protect each other, but not the clones from other chemically induced sarcomas (Algarra et al. 1991). We have data from our GR9 mouse sarcoma system indicating that the primary tumor contains multiple clones with different biological properties: H-2 positive clones that are highly immunogenic and highly metastatic, and H-2 class I negative clones with low immunogenicity and low metastatic capacity (Perez et al. 1985, 1989, 1990; Garcia-Lora et al. 2001). The enormous variety of tumor clones will interact with T lymphocytes and during the process, a "Darwinian" type of selection will take place, destroying H-2 positive tumor clones and leaving behind H-2 negative/deficient ones (Garrido et al. 2016b). An interesting observation obtained from our GR9 fibrosarcoma indicates that an H-2 class I positive tumor clone could protect against the challenge with a syngeneic H-2 class I negative clone. This suggests that a low level of antigen presentation can be sufficient to induce tumour rejection when primed T lymphocytes are available (Perez et al. 1985). A similar observation was made by Porgador and coworkers in experiments with IFN-treated B16-F10 melanoma cells (Porgador et al. 1991).

HLA-I heterogeneity or presence of both HLA-I positive and negative tumor cells in the same tumor tissue samples was also confirmed by immunohistological examination. In some cryopreserved tissue sections the expression of tumor HLA-I can be homogeneously positive or negative (see Fig. 2.3a–c). These three HLA-I staining patterns could represent three different stages of tumor development, a transition from HLA-I positive tumor at early stages (Fig. 2.3a) to HLA-I heterogeneous tumor (Fig. 2.3b), and finally to HLA-I negative tumor at more advanced late stages (Fig. 2.3c) (Aptsiauri et al. 2018). The "HLA and Cancer" component of the XII International Histocompatibility Workshop (XII IHW) that took place in Paris in 1996 classified tumor tissue sections as "positive" when more than 75% of cells were stained, heterogeneous when the positivity is between 25% and 75% and negative when there is less than 25% of positive cells (Garrido et al. 1997a, b). The work reported by Louise Koopman in a series of primary cervical carcinomas analyzing HLA expression by flow cytometry clearly indicated that HLA-I heterogeneity was also present in Papilloma Virus (HPV) induced tumors (Koopman et al. 2000).

My current interpretation is that T-cell mediated immune response induced by the host is responsible for the selection of HLA-I deficient tumor variants and that HLA-I positive, heterogeneous and negative tumor tissues represent an early and late phases of the selection (Campoli et al. 2002; Khong and Restifo 2002). Indeed, it has been reported by different groups including ourselves that the number of T cells infiltrating the tumor mass correlates with the number of HLA-I positive tumor cells, namely more HLA, more T cells and viceversa (Ryschich et al. 2005; Kikuchi et al. 2007; Aptsiauri et al. 2018).

2.1.2 Altered HLA-I Tumor Phenotypes

The complexity of the HLA system with different genetic loci and many different alleles makes difficult the characterization of the altered HLA-I phenotypes that appear during tumor progression. We reported years ago that there are several major altered HLA-I profiles that could be seen in primary tumors (Garrido et al. 1995, 1997a, b; Garrido and Algarra 2001). We classified them as follows (Fig. 2.4):

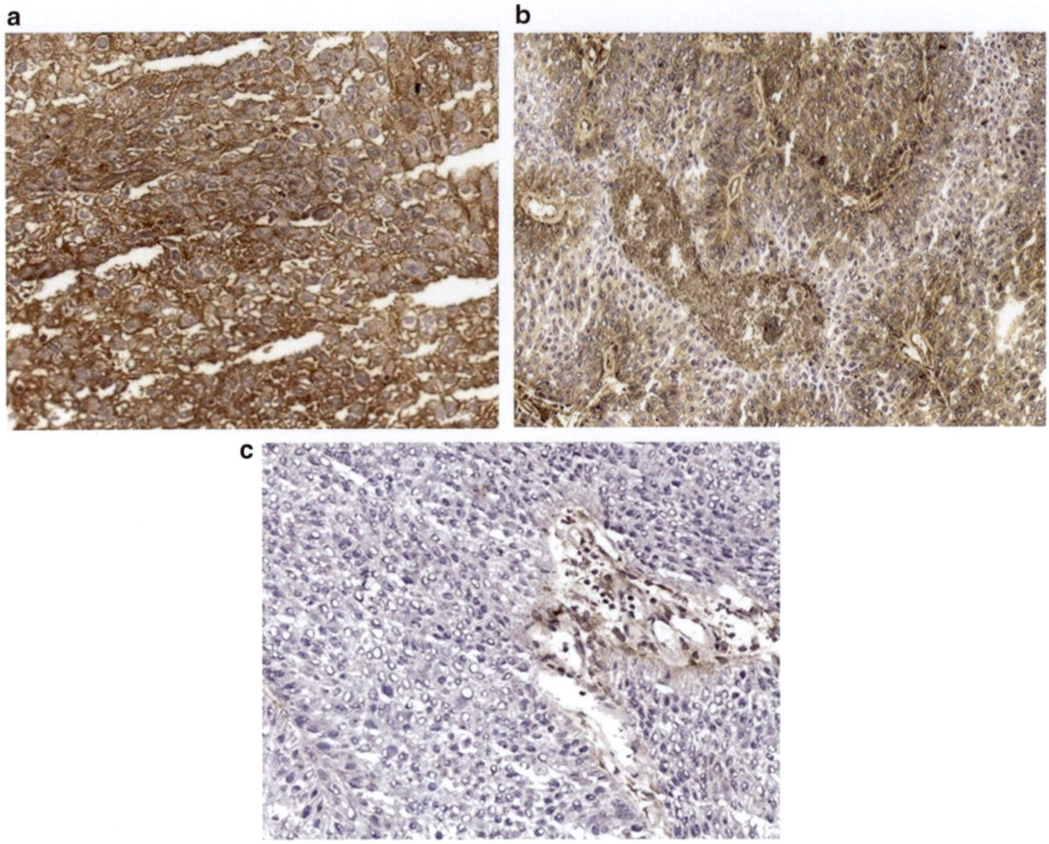

Fig. 2.3 (**a**, **b** and **c**) **Homogeneous, heterogeneous and negative HLA-I expression in human tumors.** Homogeneously positive (**a**), heterogeneous (**b**) and homogeneously negative staining of HLA class I (**c**) in different bladder carcinoma samples using the w6/32 MoAb that recognizes a conformational monomorphic epitope between the HLA-I heavy chain and the β2 microglobulin at the cell surface

***Tumor Phenotype n° I*.-HLA Class I Total Loss**

Tumor cells can lose all of the six HLA-I alleles presented in normal cells, (Fig. 2.4). We define this phenotype as n°I or HLA-I total loss, which is characterized by the absence of HLA-A, B and C loci, which produces totally negative tumor immunolabeling pattern. The surrounded stroma is positively immunolabeled and is routinely used as an internal positive control (Fig. 2.5). This phenotype has been described in different types of cancer with variable frequency and different underlying molecular mechanisms.It has been reported in 15% of melanoma and colorectal cancers and in up to 40–50% in breast, bladder or prostate carcinomas.

In melanoma and in MSI-H colorectal carcinoma around 15% of the tumor samples have this phenotype, which is caused by the absence of β2 microglobulin due to the loss of heterozigosity in chromosome 15 (LOH-15) and a mutation in the second allele of the β2m gene (Paschen et al. 2003; del Campo et al. 2014). Similar mechanisms have been reported in B-cell lymphomas (Challa-Malladi et al. 2011). I recommend reading the review by Bernal et al. 2012 that summarizes the different β2m gene mutations/deletions described in different tumors. In MSS colorectal cancer the molecular mechanisms appears to be different and caused by a LMP7/TAP2 downregulation (Cabrera et al. 2003a). In breast and prostate carcinoma total HLA-I loss is observed in more than 50% of tumor samples analyzed

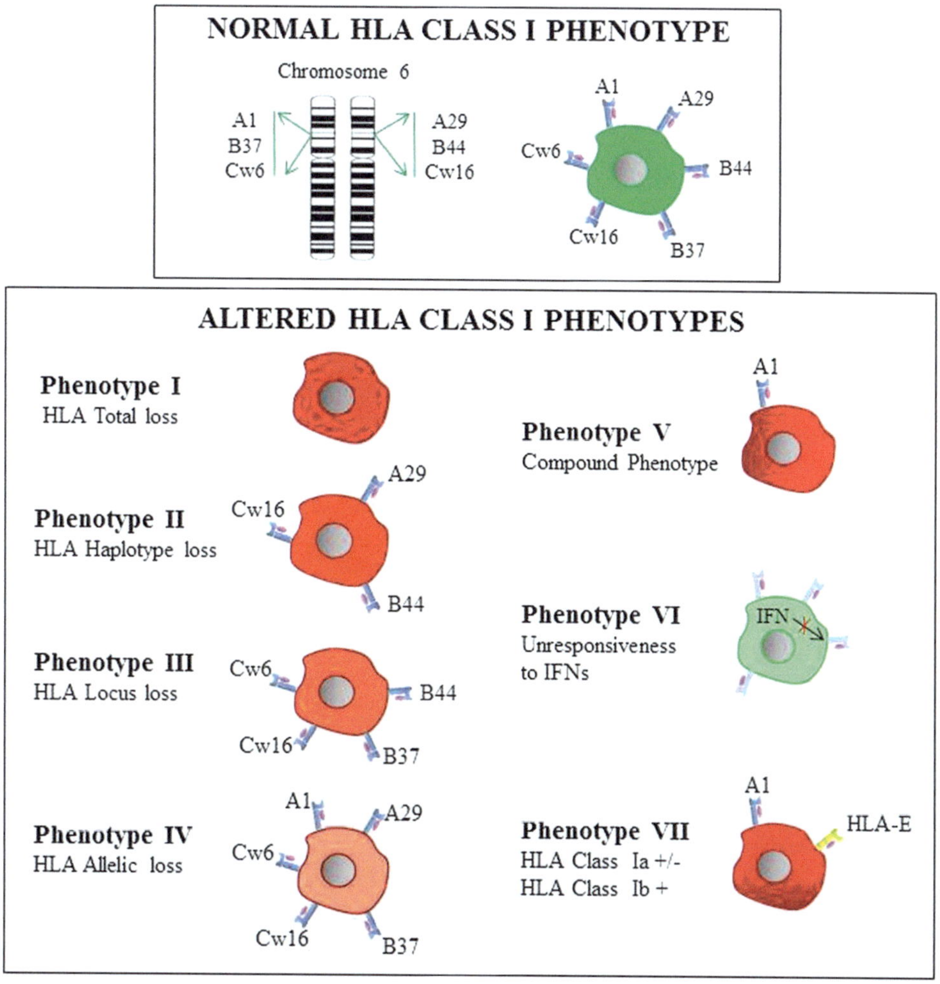

Fig. 2.4 Altered HLA class I phenotypes in human tumors. Normal somatic cells express six HLA-I alleles. Tumor cells can loose the expression of all six alleles (Ph n°I) or only one HLA haplotype and expressing only single HLA-A, B and C allele of each type (Ph n°II). Cancer cells can also experience a coordinated downregulation of the gene transcription of HLA-A, B or C locus products (Ph n°III) or loose only one HLA-I allele (Ph n°IV). In addition, there a phenotypes that combines two or more different mechanisms at the same time producing compound phenotypes (Ph n° V). There is another phenotype when tumor cells fail to upregulate HLA class I in response to IFNs (Ph n°VI). Some HLA-ABC deficient tumor cells are reported to express non classical HLA-I molecules that help to escape NK cell responses (Ph n°VII). All these phenotypes can be produced by different molecular mechanisms, some of which can be reversed by cytokines. (Garcia-Lora et al. 2003a, b, c; Garrido et al. 2010b)

(Cabrera et al. 1996; Carretero et al. 2016; Garrido et al. 2018). In prostate, bladder and lung carcinomas HLA-I total loss is associated with a coordinated transcriptional downregulation of APM and HLA-I/β2m genes (Romero et al. 2005; Carretero et al. 2016; Perea et al. 2017). This HLA tumor phenotype (Ph n°I) was the first described many years ago with the anti HLA-I monoclonal antibody that recognize a common monomorphic determinant of all HLA-I alleles formed by a conformational epitope of the heavy chain chain and the β2 microglobulin (the widely used w6/32 monoclonal antibody) (Parham et al. 1979). Later, monoclonal antibodies against β2 microglobulin light chain became available. The Daudi cell line derived from a Burkitt lymphoma

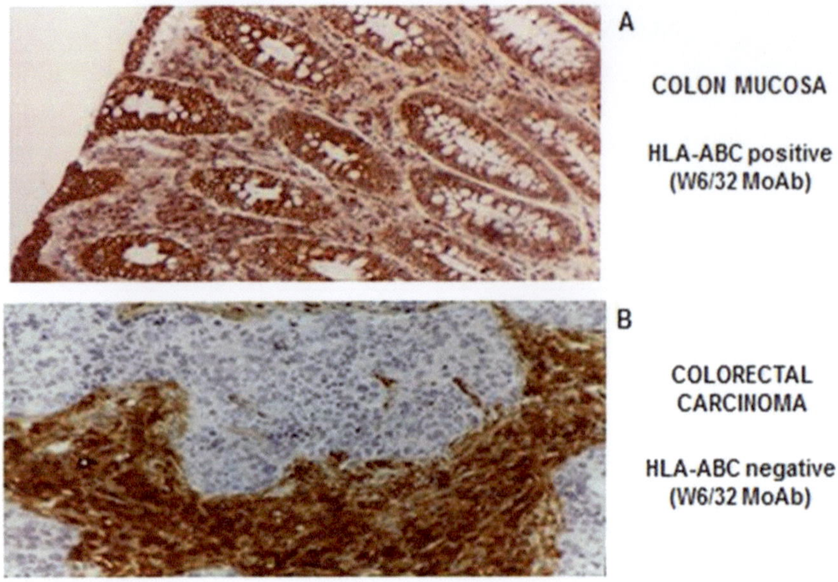

Fig. 2.5 HLA class I total loss (Ph n°I) detected in a colorectal carcinoma. The colon mucosa is HLA class I positive (**a**). The tumor parenquima is HLA-I negative and the surrounded stroma is HLA-I positive (**b**). The monoclonal antibody w6/32 recognize a monomorphic determinant (heavy chain + β2m) present in all HLA-I molecules. (Reprinted by permission from Elsevier: Aptsiauri et al. 2007)

was the first cell line reported to have a β2 microglobulin gene mutation (Rosa et al. 1983).

As mentioned earlier, this HLA-I altered phenotype can be produced by: (a) a structural/irreversible "hard" genetic alteration affecting both β2 microglobulin genes (point mutation or deletions of large DNA segments in chromosome 15 (Perez et al. 1999; Bernal et al. 2012a, b) or (b) by a transcriptional downregulation of the HLA-I, β2m or APM genes (Seliger et al. 2002). This regulatory "soft" alteration can be corrected *in vitro* by different cytokines. DNA hypermethylation of HLA class I genes have been also reported in melanoma and esophageal carcinoma as a mechanism that produces HLA-I total loss that can be reversed by 5′aza-deoxycytidine treatment (Serrano et al. 2001; Nie et al. 2001). An MHC class I transactivator (NLRC5) have been recently identified to regulate the coordinated expression of class I, LMP2/LMP7, TAP1 and β2 microglobulin genes and, therefore, is a target for immune evasion (Yoshihama et al. 2016). Similarly, tumour suppressor Fhit can positively regulate MHC class I expression on cancer cells by transcriptional regulation of class I, β2m and APM machinery genes (Romero et al. 2012).

***Tumor Phenotype n° II*.-HLA Haplotype Loss** Tumor cells can lose an HLA haplotype or one set of HLA genes (A,B & C) localized in one chromosome 6. In fact, tumor cells might loose one entire chromosome six or only part of it due to a macro or microdeletion in the short arm that carries the HLA region (Fig. 2.6). The criteria and molecular strategies to define HLA haplotype loss in human tumors were defined in my laboratory in cooperation with Marcel Tilanus from Utrech (Ramal et al. 2000a, b; Feenstra et al. 2000). This molecular mechanism occurs at early stages of tumor development and has been reported in about 30–40% of different types of malignancies, including bladder (Maleno et al. 2006), cervix (Koopman et al. 1998, 2000), colorectal (Maleno et al. 2004a, b), prostate (Carretero et al. 2016), lung (Perea et al. 2017, 2018), head and neck (Feenstra et al. 2000), melanoma (Rodriguez et al. 2005), pancreatic (Torres et al. 1996), and laryngeal carcinoma

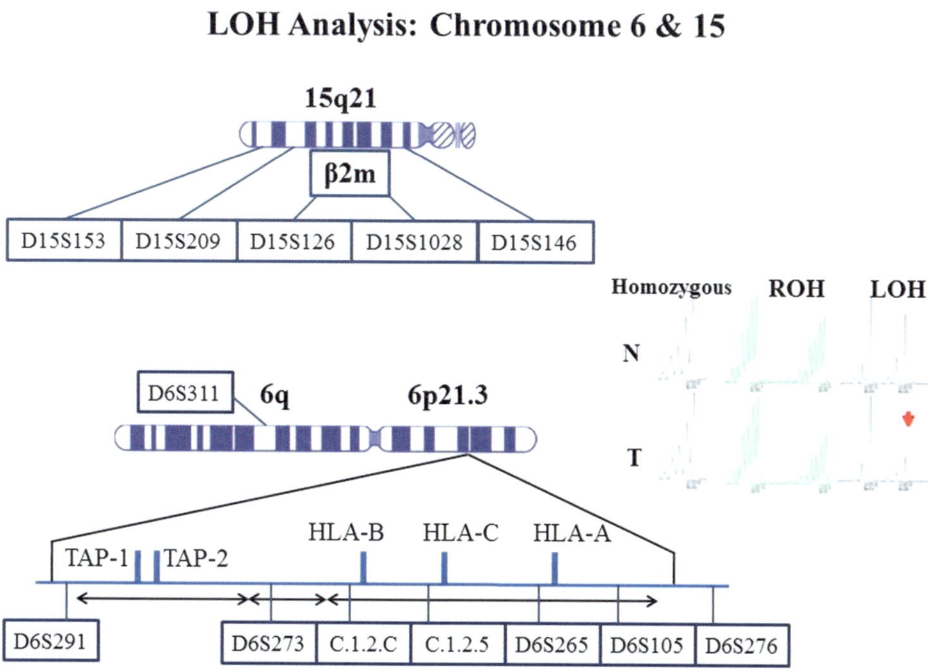

Fig. 2.6 **The analysis of Loss of heterozygosity (LOH) at the HLA and β2 microglobulin region at chromosomes 6 and 15**. The figure shows the different microsatellites used to define the LOH and provides with three examples of homozygosity (H), retention of homozygosity (ROH) and loss of homozygosity (LOH). *N* normal tissue, *T* microdissected tumor tissue

(Maleno et al. 2002), and glioblastoma (Yeung et al. 2013).

The designation of HLA haplotype loss requires DNA extraction from laser-capture microdisected parenquima to avoid contamination with DNA from the tumor stroma. We have reported that chromosome 6 loss is the most frequent mechanism producing an HLA haplotype loss in human tumors (Jimenez et al. 1999). It has been reported that chromosome loss with a simultaneous duplication and recombination contribute to the loss of heterozygosity "in vitro" (de Nooij-van Dalen et al. 1998). To analyze the presence of LOH we use amplification of different "short tandem repeat, (STRs)" or "microsatellite markers" spanning chromosome 6p in the HLA region and 6q (Fig. 2.6). Often a duplication of the remaining chromosome masks the loss of heterozygosity, which in that case can be detected by a direct HLA typing using DNA isolated from microdissected tumor tissue. It has been suggested that this HLA altered phenotype is highly malignant since these tumor cells can escape T cell mediated responses by losing one HLA-A, B and C allele, including the T cell restriction element, and at the same time, they express the remaining haplotype with another set of HLA-A, B and C genes with the ability to inhibit NK cells. Interestingly, in colorectal carcinoma "partial" HLA-I downregulation but not a "complete" loss has been linked to a poor prognosis (Watson et al. 2006). This altered HLA-I phenotype is "irreversible" or "hard" since HLA expression cannot be recovered by cytokines and only can be restored by wild type HLA-I gene transfer (Garrido et al. 2010a; Carretero et al. 2017). This altered HLA phenotype frequenty remains undetected if anti-HLA-I monoclonal antibodies against monomorphic determinants are used. It can appear together with other genetic lesions such as β2-microglobulin mutations as it has been reported in melanoma (Benitez et al. 1998; del Campo et al. 2014). HLA haplotype loss is therefore an important molecular

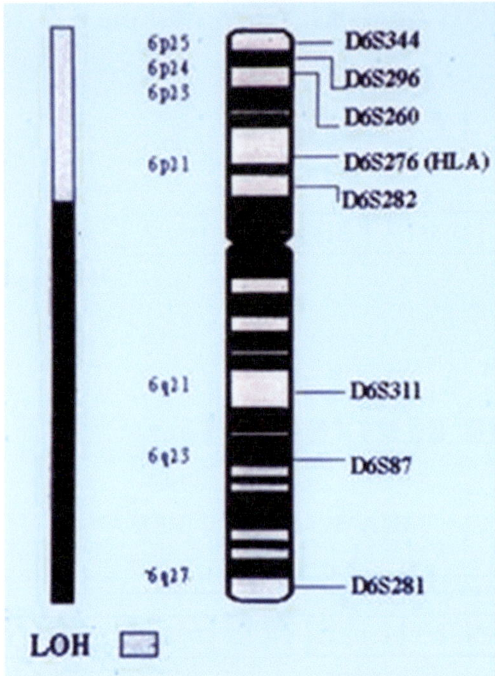

Fig. 2.7 **Loss of heterozigocity (LOH) at chromosome 6, which includes the HLA region.** This is a molecular mechanism that results in the loss of one set of HLA genes (one HLA-A,B and C haplotype). It is an early event in the "Natural History" of tumor development and can be found in a large variety of tumors.This figure depicts a macrodeletion in the 6p region of chromosome 6, which includes the entire HLA region. (Reprinted with permission of Wiley: Real et al. 1998)

mechanism in different types of tumors and leads to the loss of three different HLA class I genes (A, B and C) (Fig. 2.7). We have evidence that this is an early event in melanoma that occurs in the primary tumor, which at later stages can accumulate other defects, such as point mutations in the β2 microglobulin gene generating a phenotype n°I, or total HLA loss (del Campo et al. 2014). The same phenotype can be also produced by a combination of early LOH and dowregulation of HLA-I gene transcription, as it frequently takes place in lung carcinoma (Perea et al. 2017).

***Tumor Phenotype n° III*.-HLA-A, B or C Locus Downregulation**

Tumors can coordinately downregulate HLA-A, B or C locus-specific products producing a phenotype with only four HLA-I alleles (Fig. 2.4) (Versteeg et al. 1989; Schrier et al. 1991; Garrido et al. 1997a, b). In this case, the expression of HLA-A, B or C genes is switched off on a transcriptional level, but can be restored by IFN-γ or other Th1-type cytokines. Low expression of transcriptional factors that bind locus-specific DNA motifs can induce HLA-B locus downregulation (Soong and Hui 1992). In melanoma, a selective HLA-B locus downregulation has been reported to correlate with increased c-myc transcription (Versteeg et al. 1989; Schrier et al. 1991). The definition of this altered phenotype in tumor tissues requires the use of anti-HLA-A, B and C locus-especific monoclonal antibodies. In addition to the HLA-ABC locus specific transcriptional control of class I molecule expression, the Antigen Presentation Machinery Genes (APM) genes, including TAP1,TAP2, LMPs , are also transcriptionaly regulated and different tumors can loose or downregulate HLA-I expression by inhibiting the APM machinery (Garcia-Lora et al. 2003a, b, c; Seliger et al. 2000; Seliger 2012). Sometimes MHC heavy chain, β2 microglobulin and APM machinery genes are coordi-

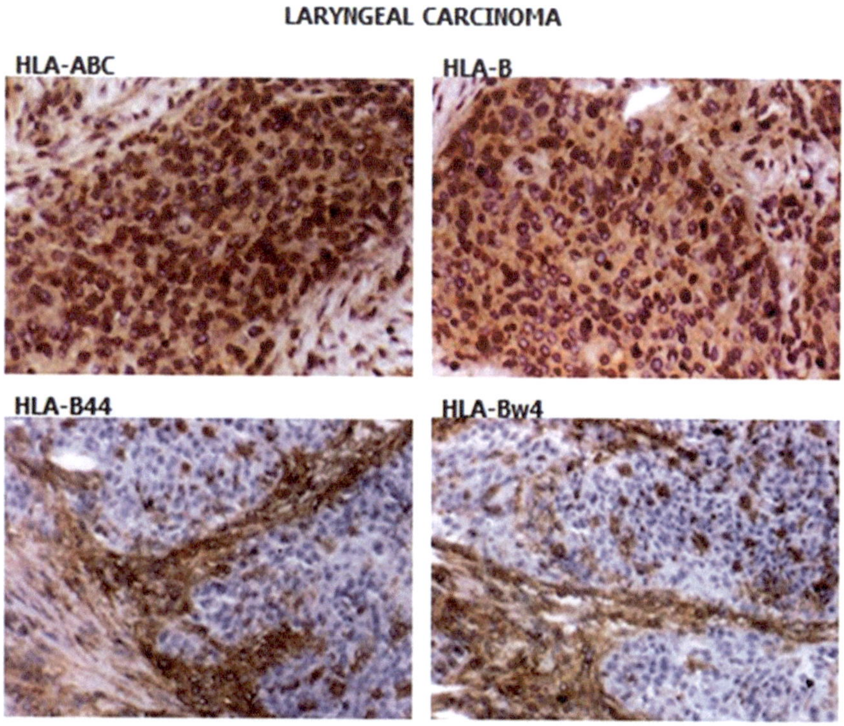

Fig. 2.8 **Loss of a single HLA-I allele in a laryngeal carcinoma (Ph n° IV).** This tumor reacted positively with MoAbs against monomorphic and locus especific HLA-I determinants (HLA ABC and HLA B). However, tumor immunolabeling was negative when we used antibody that recognizes HLA-B44 allele present in this patient's HLA genotype or with an antibody against the HLA-Bw4 associated epitope, suggesting that the B44 allele was absent on tumor cell surface

nately downregulated and produce an HLA class I total loss (Phenotype n°I). According to our published reports, these "reversible/soft" molecular mechanisms causing HLA alterations generating phenotypes n° I and III, represent approximately 1/3 of all the altered tumor phenotypes in solid tumors and cell lines. Nevertheless, more detailed studies are necessary to confirm these numbers.

***Tumor Phenotype n° IV*.-HLA Allelic Loss**

In some cases tumors lose just one single HLA-I allele out of the six expressed by somatic cells (Fig. 2.4). Mutations in HLA class I genes produce loss of the cell surface expression of one single HLA-A, B or –C allele. It has been described in a variety of human tumors and cell lines (Cabrera et al. 2003a, c, d). In solid tumours it is required to use anti-HLA monoclonal antibodies that recognize a single HLA class I gene product. Monoclonal antibodies recognizing HLA-I monomorfic determinants will give a positive reaction even in case of selective loss of a single allele (see Fig. 2.8). The identification of this altered HLA tumor phenotype is sometimes impossible due to the lack of the suitable monoclonal antibody recognizing a particular HLA-I specificity. Immunoprecipitation with the w6/32 MoAb and isoelectric focusing have been used in the past to detect single allelic losses in cell lines (Ruiz-Cabello et al. 1991a; Real et al. 1998). There have been various publication describing allelic losses in different tumor cell lines, including colorectal carcinoma cell line "LS411" with a chromosomal breakpoint in the HLA A11 allele (Browning et al. 1996); melanoma cell lines 624 MEL28, SK-MEL-29.1.22 and SK-MEL-29.1.29

with loss of the HLA-A2 allele (Wang et al. 1998, 1999); cervical cancer cell lines "CC11" with a G/T substitution in exon 2 of HLA A24 and "CSCC7" with a TGGG insertion at codon 32 in exon 2 of HLA B15 (Koopman et al. 1998, 1999); "808" cell line with a CAG/TAG substitution in exon 3 of HLA-A2 and "778" cell line with a point mutation (G/C) at the 3′acceptor site of intron 1 in HLA-A2 (Brady et al. 2000; Serrano et al. 2000). A nucleotide insertion in exon 4 has been determined to be responsible for the absence of expression of an HLA-A 0301 allele in a prostate carcinoma cell line (Jimenez et al. 2001). A single HLA-I allele loss can be sufficient to escape a particular T cell response against a tumor when the restriction element presenting the "strong tumor rejection antigen" is missing. At the same time, this phenotype provides an escape route from NK cells as the remaining HLA-B and C alleles act as inhibitory signals for KIRs. In this context, as we mentioned earlier, partial HLA-I downregulation, but not a complete loss, correlates with a poor prognosis in colorectal cancer (Watson et al. 2006).

***Tumor Phenotype n° V.*-Compound HLA Phenotype**

This is a frequent phenotype when more than one molecular mechanism contribute to the generation of the aberrant HLA-I expression accumulating different types of HLA-I alterations simultaneously during cancer progression. For instance, some tumor cells can express only an HLA-A allele on the cell surface as a result of a combination of an HLA haplotype loss (Phenotype II) produced by LOH at chromosome 6 and HLA-B and C locus transcriptional downregulation (Phenotype III) (Fig. 2.4). We described this phenotype in 1997 analyzing two melanoma cell lines (FM 55-R22 and FM 37) in a cooperative work with Dr Jesper Zeuthen from the Danish cancer Center in Copenhagen. These cell lines express only HLA-A1 and HLA-A3, respectively (Real et al. 1998). A similar finding was reported by Ikeda and coworkers in a melanoma cell line (Ikeda et al. 1997). Other groups described a cervical carcinoma cell line, which expressed only HLA-A24 allele (Brady et al. 2000; Koopman et al. 2000). In this context, we recently reported that HLA haplotype loss together with a transcriptional downregulation of HLA-A, B and C genes is a common mechanism responsible for a total HLA class I loss in approximately 60% of studied small cell lung carcinoma samples (Perea et al. 2017). This compound HLA-I phenotype that combines two o more molecular mechanisms is probably a very frequent one.

***Tumor Phenotype n° VI.*-Unresponsiveness to IFN**

IFN-γ secretion by cytotoxic T cells can induce tumour HLA-I upregulation and is critical for tumor rejection. Tumors can escape T-cell recognition by developing strategies affecting the ability to upregulate HLA-I molecules. Among them, the mutations of genes involved in IFNγ or IFNα signaling pathways have been described in different tumor cell lines (Seliger et al. 2008). The resistance to IFN can be functionally analyzed in tumor cell lines, but the frequency of this defect in human solid tumor tissues is not known. In gastric carcinoma AGS we found that total unresponsiveness to both type of IFN is associated with a low level of the transcriptional factor binding to an IFN responsive sequence element (Abril et al. 1996, 1998). In renal cell carcinoma Caki-2 resistance to IFNs is caused by the absence of DNA binding activity for IFN regulatory element factor-1 and activator of transcription Stat-1 (Dovhey et al. 2000). A recent large study demonstrated that around 25% of melanoma tumors tissue don´t display IFN mediated upregulation of HLA-I molecules (Sucker et al. 2017).

***Tumor Phenotype n° VII.*-Absence of Classical HLA-A,B,C and Aberrant Expression of HLA-Ib Molecules**

HLA E, F and G are "non Classical" class I molecules coded also by genes within the HLA region. HLA-G is characterized by limited polymorphism and the distribution restricted mainly to the extravillous trophoblast of human placenta that do not express HLA-A or B (Kovats et al. 1990; Loke and King 1991; Loke et al. 1999; Blaschitz et al. 1997). This peculiar HLA class I tissue distribution is presumed to play an important role in maintaining an immunologically privileged site where the fetus is protected from the maternal immune response in a semi-allogeneic environment. An attractive hypothesis is that tumors can use this strategy to avoid both T and NK cell responses by aberrantly expressing non classical HLA-Ib molecules in conjunction with the absence of the classical ones (HLA-Ia) (Fig. 2.4). This HLA-I tumor phenotype enables cancer cells to escape CTL responses by loosing the specific restriction element (HLA-A,B,C) and at the same time render tumor cells resistant to NK lysis by engaging HLA-Ib (HLA-G,E) molecules with NK inhibitory receptors (Garrido et al. 1997a, b; Algarra et al. 2004; De Kruijf et al. 2010). However the results reported originally in melanoma by Paul and coworkers (Paul et al. 1998) are controversial and different groups have obtained convincing data showing that HLA-G is not express at the cell surface neither in solid tumors nor in tumor cell lines (Real et al. 1999a, b; Davies et al. 2001; Pangault et al. 1999; Frumento et al. 2000).

HLA-E is a class I molecule ubiquitously transcribed in most human tissues. However a post transcriptional control may be responsible for the absence or weak expression of HLA-E at the cell surface. HLA-E binds the leader sequence peptides of newly synthesized HLA-Ia and HLA-G molecules within the endoplasmic reticulum and interacts with the NK inhibitory receptor CD94/NKG2A (Braud et al. 1997; Llano et al. 1998). In the absence of these peptides HLA-E is degraded in the endoplasmic reticulum. We observed that the cell surface expression of HLA-E in tumor cell lines is rare and correlate with downregulation of classical HLA-Ia molecules (Marin et al. 2003). An example of a melanoma metastasis expressing a single HLA-A1 allele and HLA-E is presented in Fig. 2.4. This altered HLA-I phenotype will be further discussed in the chapter "Non classical HLA class I molecules in tumors".

2.1.3 The Transition from HLA-I Positive to HLA-I Negative Tumors Induced by T Cell Immune Selection: Impact on Tumor Tissue Architecture

Tumors are originally HLA class I positive since they derive from HLA-I positive normal epithelia. We have evidences that the change of HLA-I positive to HLA-I heterogeneous or negative tumors occurs in primary tumor lesions and is directly related with the degree of infiltration by different types of T lymphocytes and other mononuclear cells such as M1 macrophages. Tumor tissue architecture changes dramatically with HLA-I loss during cancer progression (Perea et al. 2017; Garrido et al. 2017; Aptsiauri et al. 2018). When a tumor is HLA-I positive or heterogeneous, it is infiltrated with lymphocytes and macrophages owing to an immune-permissive tumor microenvironment (TME) (Permisive phase I). HLA-I positive tumor cells are actively killed by CTLs in phase I, leading to a progressive T cell immune selection of HLA-I deficient tumor cells (Encapsulated Phase II) (see Fig. 2.9). Tumour infiltration by T lymphocytes (TILs) and by other immune cells has been described long time ago by pathologists, but has never been directly and clearly linked to the destruction of HLA-I positive and selection of HLA-I negative tumour cells (Galon et al. 2006; Salgado et al. 2015). Oncogenic viruses and activation of proto-oncogenes can directly downregulated MHC/HLA class I antigens whithout a direct involvement of T lymphocytes in some tumors like cervical and breast carcinomas (Bartholomew et al. 1997; Bernards et al. 1986).

Phase II is characterized by the lack of tumor infiltrating cells and a clear separation between HLA-I negative tumor and HLA-I positive stroma cells. It is very likely that due to the low cytotoxic activity of CD8+ T lymphocytes and the absence of natural killer (NK) cells, the host is trying to isolate tumor cells from the rest of the body while tumor cells are actively creating an immunosuppressive microenvironment by inducing stromal reorganization and generation of a structure similar to a Th2 granuloma. As a result, tumor archi-

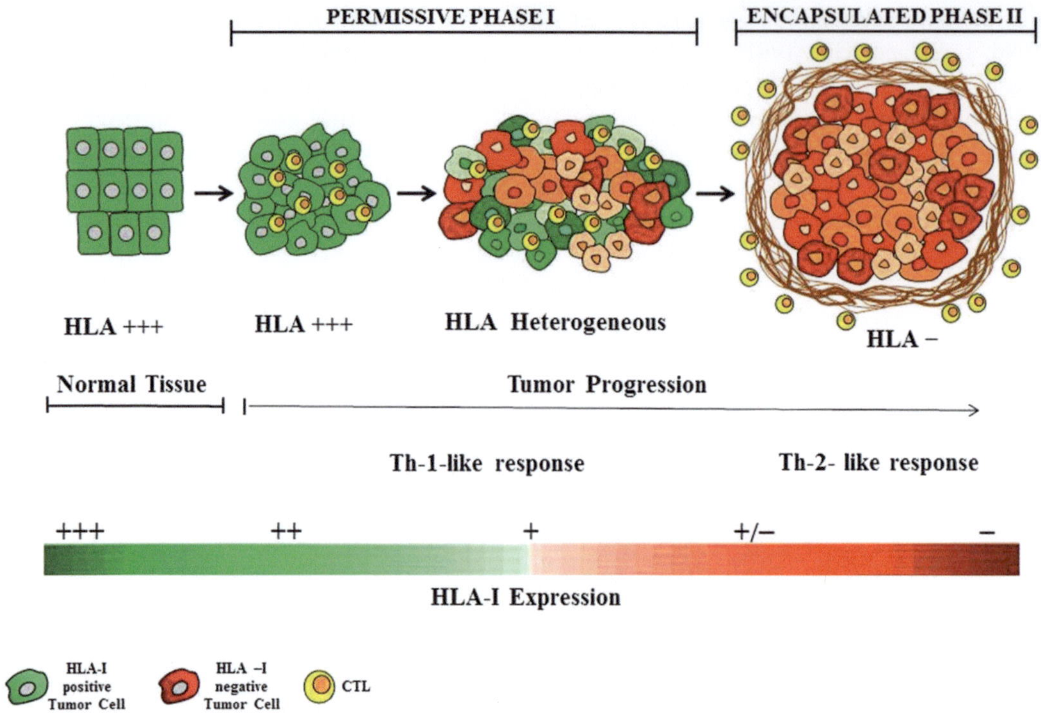

Fig. 2.9 **The transition from HLA class-I positive to HLA-I heterogeneous and, finally, to HLA class I negative primary tumors.** Tumors derive from HLA-I positive normal tissues and remain HLA class I positive at early stages of tumor development. Tumor cells are infiltrated by T cells (permissive phase I). Later, the HLA-I expression is heterogeneous with an enormous variety of tumour cell clones expressing different amount of HLA class I molecules. HLA-I deficient cells are immunoselected resulting in a tumor composed only of homogenously HLA-I negative cells surrounded by a stroma-like capsule and by the different mononuclear cells including T lymphocytes (encapsulated phase II)

tecture changes, generating tumor nodes surrounded by different types of T-cells/leucocytes/macrophages and probably other elements of the tumor microenvironment, including Tregs and MDSCs. Furthermore, this phase is also characterized by a marked peritumoral localization of fibroblasts and alternatively activated macrophages providing a physical barrier and forming a "non-permissive" tissue structure. Such tumor tissue organization can be observed in a variety of tumors of different histological type, however it has not been previously associated with the absence of HLA-I expression (Garrido et al. 2017). The encapsulated HLA-I negative tumor without activated tumor infiltrating immune cells represents a condition of "Immunological Silence". This transition probably lasts for a short period of time ending with the tumor composed only of HLA-I negative cells, This is a "stand by" situation since the tumor is continuously locally growing and iniciating the complex phenomenon of invasion and metastatic colonization.

An important question raised frequently is "Why NK cells are not killing the HLA-I negative or deficient tumor cells" inside the tumor nest? We have immunohistological evidences that NK cells are outside and cannot enter the tumor nest in the encapsulated phase II (Garrido et al. 2017). There are different reports indicating that NK cells are very eficient in destroying circulating HLA-I negative tumor cells, i.e. when producing blood borne metastasis in uveal melanoma (Blom et al. 1997; Ericsson et al. 2001) and in microsatellite unstable MSH-I colorectal carcinomas (Kloor et al. 2010). NK cells despite recognizing the absence of HLA class I (Lanier 2005) remains outside the solid tumor mass. In this context, tumor cells frequently lose only partially HLA class I molecule expression i.e. one HLA haplotype or one single allele with conserved HLA B and C alleles, which can inhibit NK cell mediated cytotoxicity (see previously described HLA altered tumor phenotypes II and IV).

The following figures illustrate this transition process in lung cancer patients starting with HLA class-I positive tumor with TILs inside the tumour nests: Permissive phase I (Fig. 2.10a). This phase is followed by a heterogeneous HLA-I expression pattern as a consequence of a continuous T cell mediated immuneselection with TILs only in HLA-I positive areas (Fig. 2.10b). Finally, the T cell mediated attack ends with a tumor composed "only" of HLA class I negative cancer cells with lymphocytes in the stroma surrounding the tumor: Encapsulated Phase II (Fig. 2.10c).

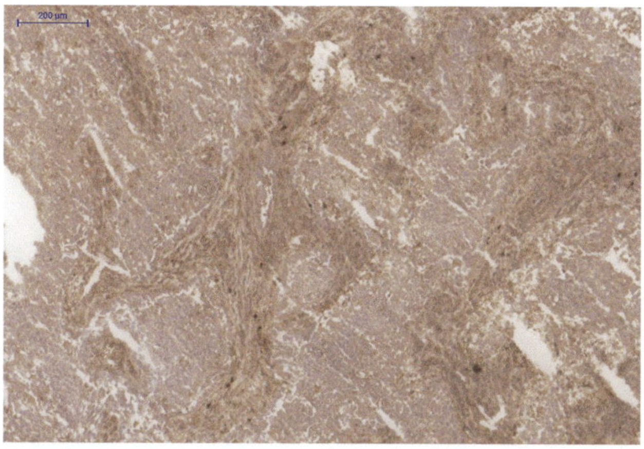

A-a.- Lung cancer tissue stained with w6/32 MoAb recognizing HLA ABC molecules. There is an homogeneously positive HLA-I expression.

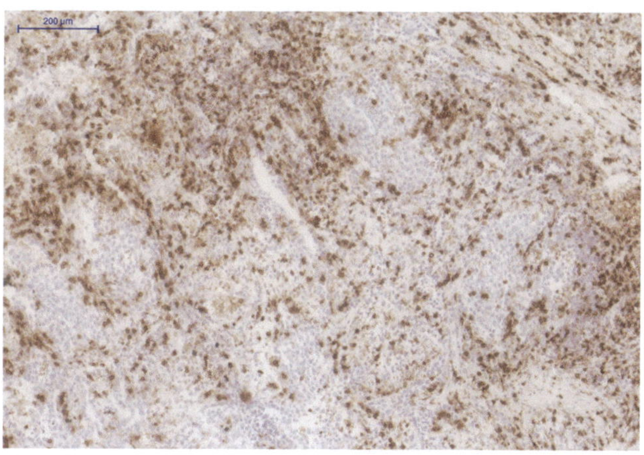

A-b.- The same tissue stained with an antibody against CD8 showing a massive intratumor infiltration with T lymphocytes.

Fig. 2.10 HLA I positive, heterogeneous and negative tumors and pattern of T cell infiltration. HLA class I expression and tumor infiltrating lymphocytes in tumor tissues from three different lung cancer patients using an antibody against a common epitope of HLA-A,B and C molecules (w6/32)(a) and an anti CD8 MoAb(b). (**a**) homogeneously positive HLA-I staining and T cell infiltration inside the tumor nest. (**b**) heterogeneous HLA-I staining with positive and negative HLA-I tumor cells and T cell infiltration only in HLA-I positive areas. (**c**) HLA-I negative tumor staining with HLA-I positive stroma and CD8 positive T cells outside the tumor nest in the stroma

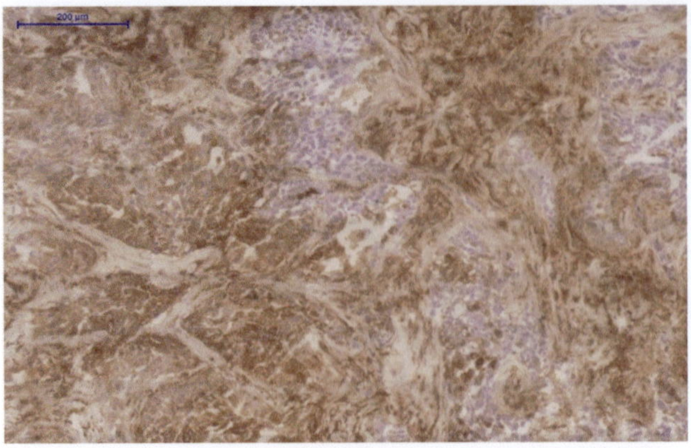

***B-a.*-** *Another lung cancer tissue showing an heterogeneous HLA I expression with positive and negative areas.*

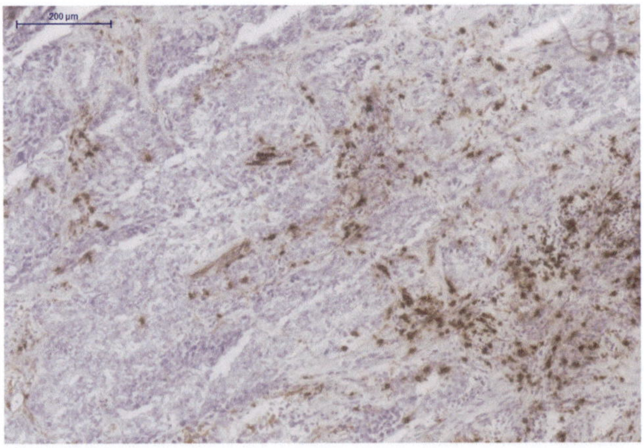

***B-b.*-** *The same cancer tissue showing presence of TILs only in HLA-I positive areas.*

Fig. 2.10 (continued)

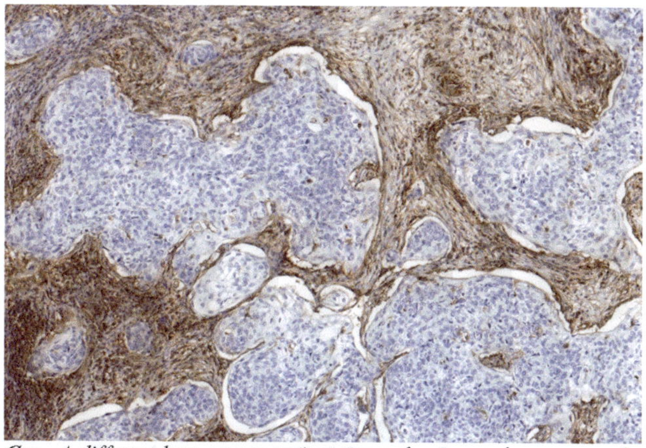

C-a.- A different lung cancer patient-tissue showing an homogeneously HLA-I negative tumor tissue surrounded by HLA-I positive stroma.

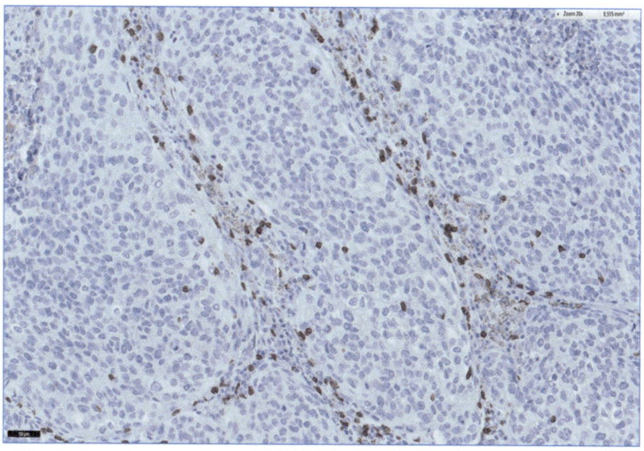

C-b.- T lymphocytes are restrained at the tumor mass margin in the stroma, without a direct contact with tumor cells.

Fig. 2.10 (continued)

2.1.4 HLA Class I Loss in Different Tumor Tissues

HLA class I losses is a general phenomenon observed in tumors derived from HLA class I positive epithelia (Natali et al. 1989; Garrido and Klein 1991a, b; Garrido et al. 1993). The analysis of HLA-I expression in different tumor tissues using microdissection as well as immunohistological and molecular techniques have provided insights into the frequency and mechanisms underlying HLA-I downregulation. The information obtained clearly indicates that **1st**: the frequency of HLA-I loss in tumors is very high, more that 90% already defined in some tumors (Fig. 2.11). An important requirement for these studies is the use of cryopreserved tumor tissues since there are only few anti HLA MoAbs that work in paraffin embedded sections and they only recognize monomorphic determinants (Cabrera et al. 2003a). Additionally, the panel of available locus and allele specific anti HLA MoAbs is still very limited. These limitations suggest that the % of HLA class I losses is still underestimated in some tumor types. **2nd**: there are shared mechanisms responsible for HLA-I loss described in different tumors. One is the loss of heterozygosity (LOH) in chromosome 6 and 15 where the HLA and β2 microglobulin genes are located (Maleno et al. 2011) **3rd**: Different molecular mechanisms can lead to the same

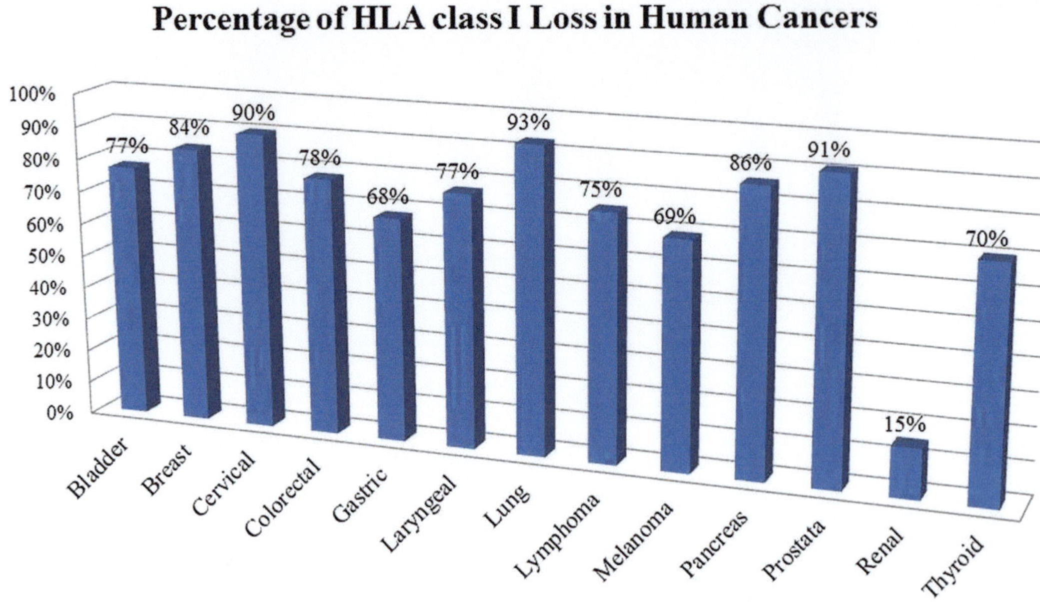

Fig. 2.11 Percentage of HLA class I loss in different human tumors. Data were obtained from immunohistological analysis of cryopreserved and paraffin embedded tumor tissues using different anti HLA-I monoclonal antibodies defining HLA class I total, HLA-I locus specific and HLA-I allelic losses reported by different laboratories

altered HLA class I phenotype (Rodriguez et al. 2007a, b) **4th:** there are peculiar molecular mechanism present in certain tumors, i.e. β2 microglobulin mutations in melanoma and MSI-H colorectal carcinoma (Bernal et al. 2012a). **5th**: In contrast, the molecular mechanism responsible for HLA class I total loss in breast and prostate carcinoma is not yet clearly defined. **6th**: there are some tumors extensively analysed for HLA expression by different research groups such as melanoma, colorectal, lung, bladder, head and neck cancer, while the information available for other tumors like gastric, pancreas, gliomas, neuroblastomas, endometrial, esophageal, basal cell carcinomas of the skin (Cabrera et al. 1992) and rhabdomiosarcomas (Fernandez et al. 1991) is still very limited. **7th:** there are reports indicating that in some tumors HLA class I expression coincides with intratumor T cell infiltration, namely more HLA-I/more T cells, favouring the idea that T cell immunoselection is playing a major role (Aptsiauri et al. 2018). This remains to be confirmed in other types of cancer. In this context, it is well stablished that some cellular or virus oncogene products can interfere with HLA-I expression like in cervical or breast tumors (Stern 1996; Koopman et al. 1998; Koopman et al. 2000; Brady et al. 2000). Figure 2.11 summarizes the % of HLA expression for different human tumors with data obtained from different laboratories. In the following sections I will be analyzing the available information on HLA class I expression in tumors derived from different tissues presented in alphabetical order.

Biliary Tract Carcinoma

Biliary tract cancer (BTC) is a rare malignancy with a poor prognosis. It can be classified into three major subtypes: Cholangiocarcinoma of intrahepatic and extrahepatic origin and gallbladder adenocarcinoma. Goeppert and coworkers showed in 2013 that tumour infiltrating T lymphocytes represent a favourable prognostic marker in extrahepatic colangiocarcinoma and gallbladder carcinoma (Goeppert et al. 2013). The HLA class I analysis of 334 BTC and 71 high grade biliary intrahepithelial lesions showed a low HLA-I expression in 48% of BTC and loss of MHC-I during the evolution from intraepithelial into invasive neoplastic lesion (Goeppert et al. 2015). In addition, this same study showed that reduced MHC-I expression in BTC is linked to a shortened overall survival. The molecular mechanim/s responsible for HLA class I losses in biliart tract tumors need to be defined in the future.

Bladder Carcinoma

The term "superficial bladder carcinoma" encompasses a spectrum of diseases that range from the innocuous Ta grade I tumor to a life-threatening grade III T1 tumor. Grade I tumors are usually papillary and are confined to the mucosal surface. It has been reported that approximately 40% of these tumors showed invasion of the lamina propia at inicial diagnosis, with a 5-year survival of up to 65%. Normal bladder mucosa expresses HLA class I antigens (Berah et al. 1970; Fleming et al. 1981; Daar et al. 1984; Levin et al. 1991; Witjes et al. 1995).

As the bladder undergoes malignant transformation to transitional cell carcinoma, several phenotypic changes can be detected on the cell surface. Among these, the loss of MHC class I molecules in normal bladder epithelia has been reported by different researchers including our group (see Fig. 2.12). Cryopreserved tumor tissues were analyzed by immunohistochemistry using a variety of MoAbs recognizing monomorphic, locus specific and allelic HLA-I determinants (Levin et al. 1991, 1992; Tomita et al. 1990; Klein et al. 1996). Moderate (grade II) and high-grade (grade III) tumors showed losses (32%) or reductions in HLA class I antigens to a much greater extent than low-grade (grade I) tumors when W6/32 mAb were used (Tomita et al. 1990).

A study of 68 tumor sections by Nouri and coworkers (Nouri et al. 1990) showed that 42% of the cases had reduced or absent expression of HLA molecules. The use of polymorphic antibodies against HLA-A2, HLA-A3, Bw4, and Bw6 increased the frequency of detected HLA-I defects to 73% (Nouri et al. 1994). A similar frequency of HLA negative expression (75%) was found also in metastasis (Cordon-Cardo et al. 1991). Our laboratory analyzed a series of bladder tumor samples and also found a high frequency of HLA class I antigen loss (85%). This % was the summatory of HLA class I total loss (Phenotype n°I) found in 45% of the samples and HLA-I allelic loss (Phenotype n° IV) (Cabrera et al. 2003a).

In 2005 we reported that in bladder cancer a coordinated downregulation of the antigen presentation machinery is responsible for HLA ABC loss (Romero et al. 2005) and is associated with a high frequency of LOH in chromosome 6p21.3 region where the HLA region is located (Maleno et al. 2006). Our results strongly suggest that a combination of two independent molecular mechanisms is responsible for the HLA-I total loss observed in 45% of bladder cancer: LOH in chromosome 6 and a coordinated transcriptional down-regulation of the antigen presentation machinery, HLA class I and β2 microglobulin genes (Maleno et al. 2006; Romero et al. 2005). These results are similar to what we recently observed in lung carcinoma. We found that HLA-I total loss in lung cancer occurs in 40% of

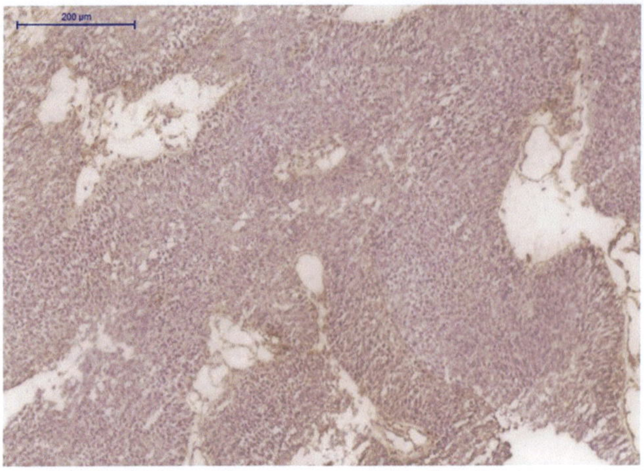

A.- PATIENT n°1.- *Homogeneous HLA class I positive staining of tumor parenquima and stroma (w6/32 MoAb).*

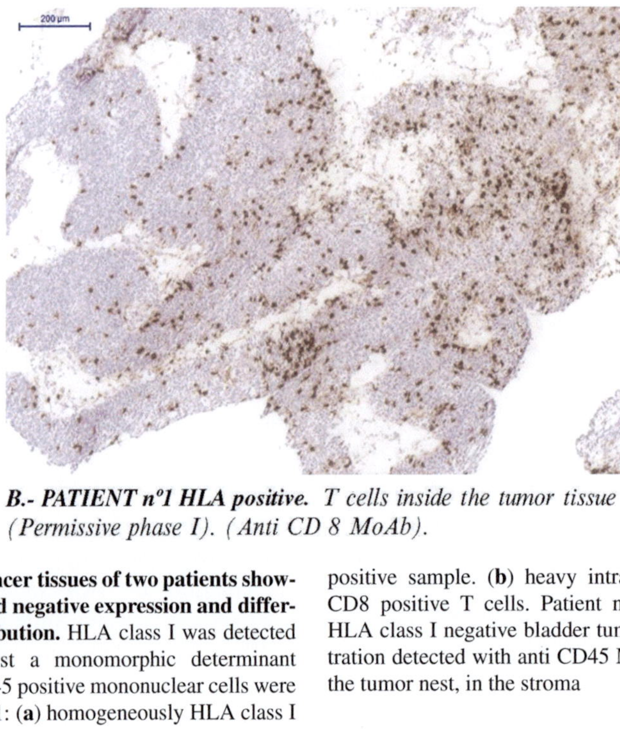

B.- PATIENT n°1 HLA positive. *T cells inside the tumor tissue (Permissive phase I). (Anti CD 8 MoAb).*

Fig. 2.12 Bladder cancer tissues of two patients showing HLA-I positive and negative expression and different lymphocyte distribution. HLA class I was detected using a MoAb against a monomorphic determinant (w6/32). CD8 and CD45 positive mononuclear cells were also stained. Patient n°1: (**a**) homogeneously HLA class I positive sample. (**b**) heavy intratumor infiltration with CD8 positive T cells. Patient n°2: (**c**) homogeneously HLA class I negative bladder tumor tissue. (**d**) The infiltration detected with anti CD45 MoAb is located outside the tumor nest, in the stroma

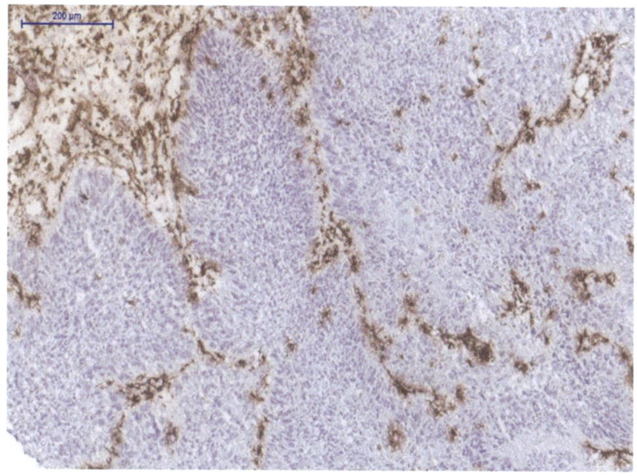

C PATIENT nº2.- HLA class I negative tumor tissue. The stroma is HLA-I positive (w6/32 MoAb).

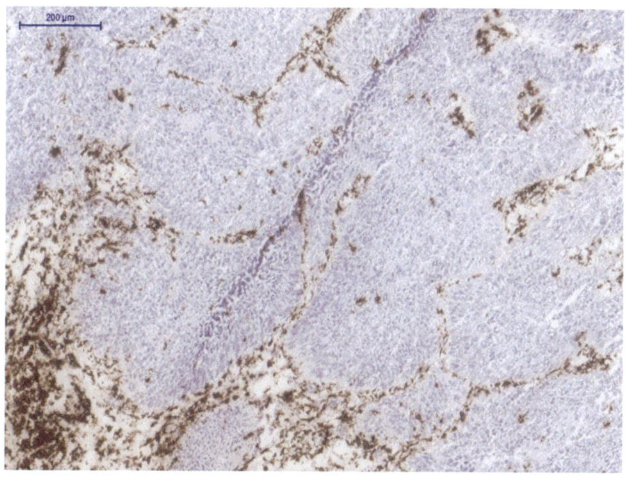

***D.- PATIENT nº2.- HLA class I negative tumor.-** The infiltrating cells are located in the stroma surounding the tumor nest, (Anti CD45 MoAb).*

Fig. 2.12 (continued)

patients and is produced by a combination of LOH in chromosome 6 and a coordinated transcriptional downregulation of HLA/β2m/APM genes (Perea et al. 2017). Interestingly, we did not find β2 microglobulin mutations in bladder and lung cancer (Romero et al. 2005; Perea et al. 2017).

An intravesicular instilation of BCG has become a major breakthrough in immunotherapy of early stage superficial bladder cancer before the basal membrane invasion. This treatment developed and proposed by Morales and coworkers (Morales et al. 1976) is still a routine treatment of bladder cancer in many hospitals all over the world with very encouraging results demonstrating the absence of cancer recurrence in about 40% of the treated patients (Kitamura et al. 2006). In this context, we have reported that the post-BCG recurrent bladder cancer lesions have increased percentage of LOH in chromosome 6 and 15 as compares to the lesions before therapy suggesting that BCG activates T cells and promotes selection of cancer cells with HLA class I loss caused by LOH in chromosome 6 (Carretero et al. 2011). In addition, more recently we obtained data confirming that tumor T-cell infiltration correlates with the number of HLA-I positive bladder cancer cells (Fig. 2.12).

Breast Carcinoma

Among breast tumors, ductal adenocarcinoma is the most common histological type of breast cancer. Proliferation of epithelial cells from galactophorous ducts may be preceded by *in situ* carcinoma, characterized by the proliferation of cells within the ducts without invasion of the basal membrane. Lobular carcinoma is the second most frequent type (5–10%). The third type of breast cancer (medullary carcinoma) is a rare entity (1%). Studies at the molecular level have demonstrated many chromosomal aberrations in breast cancer, including LOH in several chromosomes in almost all types of breast tumors (Mertens et al. 1997; Eisen and Weber 1998). Normal epithelia and low-risk proliferative lesions of the breast tissue are HLA class I positive (Garrido et al. 1993). Previous studies by different groups, including ours, have demonstrated that HLA class I antigens are downregulated in 40–50% of tumor tissues of patients diagnosed with breast carcinoma (Fleming et al. 1981; Perez et al. 1986; Natali et al. 1983a; Whitwell et al. 1984; Moller et al. 1989; Wintzer et al. 1990; Concha et al. 1991a, 1991b; Maiorana et al. 1995). Introduction of anti-HLA mAbs that recognize HLA alleles in tissue sections allowed obtaining more detailed characteristics of HLA alterations.

According to our data the frequency of various types of HLA class I alterations in breast cancer is around 88.5% (Cabrera et al. 1996; Algarra et al. 1999, 2000). In some breast cancer cell lines we observed that the level of HLA expression is influenced by steroid hormones (Rodriguez et al. 1994). A concordant downregulation of HLA class I antigen and TAP1/TAP2 staining was observed in 22% of 37% high-grade breast carcinoma lesions and complete loss of TAP2 was found in 8% of the cases (Vitale et al. 1998). Altered expression of class I, TAP, and β2 microglobulin genes at once was found in primary and metastatic breast carcinomas (Kaklamanis et al. 1995). Forty-four percent of lymph node metastases demonstrated a complete class I loss. The high incidence of HLA class I loss in breast cancer patients shows that adjuvant immunotherapy to induce HLA class I expression may be of value in a subgroup of patients with reversible HLA class I defects (Fig. 2.13). Madjd and coworkers (Madjd et al. 2005) reported that total loss of MHC class I is an independent indicator of good prognosis in breast carcinomas suggesting that NK cells might control these HLA-I negative variants during metastatic dissemination via blood circulation. In this context, MHC class I negative metastatic

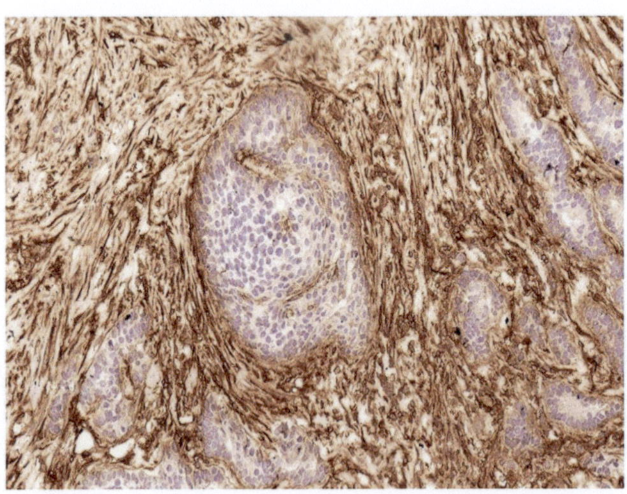

Fig. 2.13 HLA class I negative breast carcinoma. The stroma is positively stained (W6/32 MoAb)

cells from breast cancer patients have been detected in bone marrow (Zia et al. 2001).

Despite the growing evidence indicating that HLA class I downregulation in breast cancer is a frequent event, little is known about the molecular mechanism/s responsible for this aberrations. In this context, we have recently reported that LOH at chromosomes 6 and 15 that carry the HLA and β2 microglobulin genes is observed in 33 and 25%, of breast carcinoma respectively (Garrido et al. 2018). In contrast, in this same study, β2 microglobulin mutations were not detected in 25 breast cancer tissues with HLA-I total loss.

Cervical Carcinoma

Carcinoma of the cervix usually arises in the transitional zone between squamous and columnar cell epithelia. Approximately 80% of all malignant tumors of the cervix are squamous cell carcinomas, 10% are adenocarcinomas and 10% are adenoacanthomas.Three grades of premalignant lesion are recognized: cervical intraephitelial neoplasia (CIN) I, II and III. Carcinomas are staged as follows: IA; early invasive, not grossly visible; IB, IIA, IIB, IIIA confined to the cervix and IIIB, IVA, and IVB with involvement of the pelvis, bladder, and distant metastase, respectively. A crucial event in the malignant progression of CIN appears to be the upregulation of high-risk human papillomavirus (HPV) early gene expression (Stern 1996). HPV types 16 and 18 are associated with approximately 70% of all cervical carcinomas. These high-risk types of HPV are invariably detected in the moderate and severe stages of preinvasive malignancy. CIN II and III tumors of the cervix are among the most thoroughly analyzed for HLA expression (Torres et al. 1993; Keating et al. 1995; Koopman et al. 1998, 2000; Brady et al. 2000). Cervical carcinoma is associated with infection by different types of human papilloma virus in more than 99% of cases (Walboomers et al. 1999) and the well-established multistep process of carcinogenesis during the "natural history" of tumor development has provided well-characterized material for the study of MHC alterations. Cervical carcinoma is one of the tumor tissues extensively analyzed for HLA expression in which multiple molecular mechanisms have been identified that are responsible for HLA-I alterations (Koopman et al. 2000; Brady et al. 2000). Normal cervix epithelium and premalignant lesions are HLA class I positive (Garrido et al. 1993) (Fig. 2.14) and show no alteration with monomorphic, locus or allele-specific anti-HLA mAbs (Hilders et al. 1994).

On the other hand, the frequency of the loss of HLA class I expression based on Immunohistochemical analysis in cervical carcinoma is very high (Connor and Stern 1990; Keating et al. 1995; Garrido et al. 1993, 1997a) and can range from complete absence of all HLA-A, B and C alleles and β2 microglobulin to loss of expression of a single allele (Keating et al. 1995). It has been reported that more than 96% of all cervical carcinomas show some HLA class I alteration in the tumor cells and almost 70% are caused by multiple genetic alterations at chromosome 6p21.3, including genomic deletions and mutations in class I genes (Koopman et al. 1998). Four altered pheno/genotype categories have been described (Koopman et al. 2000): (1) Total HLA class I loss (10%) and retention of heterozygosity (ROH) at 6p21.3; this category includes HLA losses caused by β2 microglobulin gene mutations. (2) HLA haplotype loss (50%) caused by LOH at chromosome 6p21.3 (20–30%), wich represents a common mechanism by which HLA genes and their products are eliminated (Kersemaekers et al. 1998; Mazurenko et al. 1999; Ramal et al. 2000a). (3) B locus or HLA-A and B downregulation associated with ROH and/or allelic imbalance at 6p21.3 (10%). (4) HLA-A or -B allelic loss (17%), mostly associated with gene mutations. HLA-B antigens have been found to be more frequently downregulated than HLA-A antigens (Brady et al. 2000), suggesting that the molecular basis of this particular alteration in HLA-A and -B locus expression could be different. The relationship between the presence of high-risk HPV in cervical lesions and HLA class I downregulation has not been clearly established, but there are reports indicating that integration of high-risk HPV 16 and 18 sequences in cervix tumor DNA is linked to the downregulation of HLA class I antigens by steroid hormones

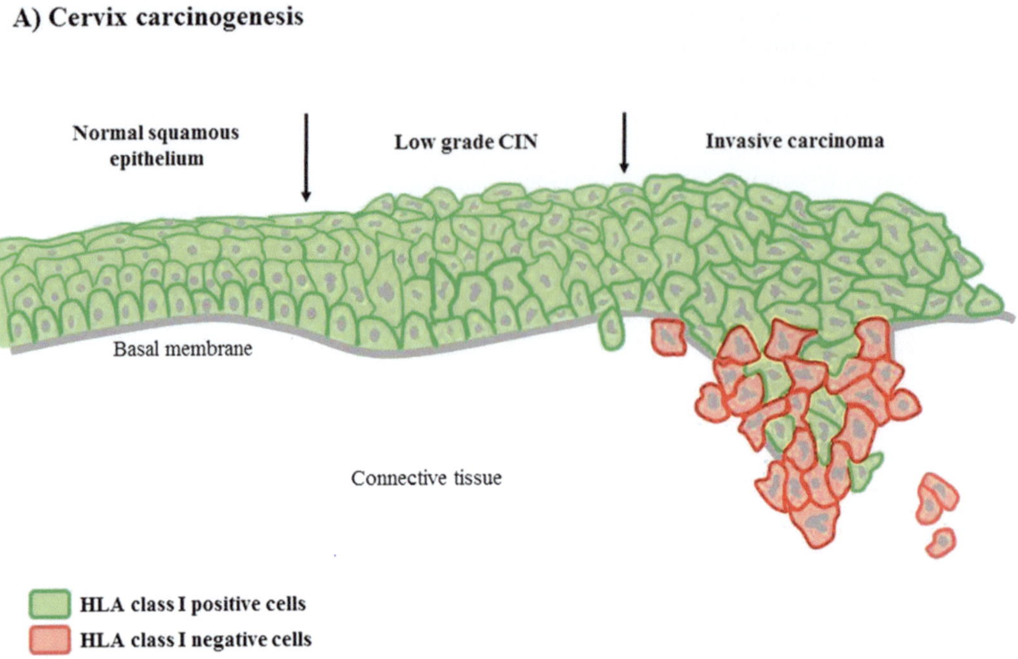

Fig. 2.14 HLA class I expression in normal mucosa, bening lesions and cervical carcinoma. The expression is positive in normal tissue and CIN lesions and negative in invasive carcinoma

(Bartholomew et al. 1997). Altered HLA expression associated with antigen processing machinery (APM) defects, including the loss of transporter protein TAP1, has been also reported (Cromme et al. 1994; Mehta et al. 2008).

Colorectal Carcinoma

Colorectal cancer is a tumor extensively studied for HLA expression. Different groups analyzed HLA in cryopreserved tumor tissues and found total as well as locus and allelic losses HLA losses in this type of malignancy (Csiba et al. 1984; Momburg et al. 1986a, b, 1989; Moore et al. 1986, 1989; Gutierrez et al. 1987; Durrant et al. 1987; Rees et al. 1988; Momburg and Koch 1989; Smith et al. 1988, 1989; Lopez-Nevot et al. 1989; Eyal et al. 1990; Kaklamanis and Hill 1992; Kaklamanis et al. 1992; Browning et al. 1993a). The transition from normal colorectal epithelium to adenoma and later to carcinoma is associated with the acquisition of different cumulative molecular events. Some key changes include loss of chromosomes 5q, 17p, and 18q and mutation in the *K-ras* oncogene (Volgelstein et al. 1988; Fearon and Volgestein 1990). Normal epithelia, as well as benign and premalignant lesions of the colon, are HLA class I positive. Although other genetic and morphological changes occur at this stage of tumor development, the expression of HLA class I antigens is apparently not altered (Garrido et al. 1993; Tsioulias et al. 1993). For instance, colon adenomas that are known to accumulate several activated protooncogens such as *K-ras* are strongly HLA class I-positive (Gutierrez et al. 1987). Early studies in colorectal carcinomas using anti-HLA mAbs directed against monomorphic HLA determinants revealed HLA class I losses in 30–40% of the tumors (Moller et al. 1991). However, when a broader panel of mAbs against monomorphic, locus-specific, and allele-specific determinants was used, the incidence of HLA losses increased up to 73% (Cabrera et al. 1998). Despite the high frequency of altered HLA expression detected in these tumors, it was not possible at that time to study all the HLA alleles suggesting that HLA-I losses were underestimated (Kaklamanis et al. 1992).

Today we know that colorectal cancer (CRC) is a heterogeneous disease that can be divided in two major groups (Kloor et al. 2010): (a) 15% of CRC are hypermutated with microsatellite instability (MSI-high) because of a defect in the DNA mismatch repair (MMR) system and ubiquitous somatic mutations in repeated DNA sequences that occur during colon carcinogenesis (Ionov et al. 1993); they might develop sporadically or in the context of the hereditary nonpolyposis colorectal cancer (HNPCC) or Lynch syndrome (Kloor et al. 2007); and (b) 85% of CRC belong to the non mutated- microsatellite stable (MSS) group (Kloor and von Knebel Doeberitz 2016). These two groups of CRC also have different molecular mechanism responsible for HLA class I alterations (Jimenez et al. 2000; Cabrera et al. 2003a). In the former, inactivation of the β2 microglobulin gene is responsible for HLA-I total loss (Browning et al. 1996; Kloor et al. 2005), and in the second type, a transcriptional dowregulation of LMP7 and TAP2 genes account for HLA-I alterations (Cabrera et al. 2003a) associated with a high frequency of HLA haplotype loss (Maleno et al. 2004a, b, 2011). Complete loss of expression of HLA class I antigens in MSI-H colorectal tumors is associated with a lack of β2 microglobulin synthesis or with the synthesis of truncated β2 microglobulin (Bicknell et al. 1996; Kloor et al. 2007; Bernal et al. 2012a, b). Any genetic or posttranslational event that impairs β2 microglobulin production results in failure to form peptide-heavy chain-β2 microglobulin complexes on the cell surface (Browning et al. 1996; Cabrera et al. 1998). This was observed in a series of MSI-H colorectal tumors in which the absence of HLA class I expression was associated with mutations in β2 microglobulin gene (Browning et al. 1996; Bicknell et al. 1994).

We have evidence that LOH in chromosomes 6 and 15 affecting the HLA region and the β2 microglobulin gene is a frequent event in MSS-colorectal cancer (Maleno et al. 2004a, b, 2011), and most likely is an early event in CRC tumor development (Bernal et al. 2012a, b). We analyzed β2 microglobulin gene in 31 MSS tumors (out of 162 cases) with HLA class I total loss and did not find β2 microglobulin mutations suggesting that other mechanisms are involved in the generation of HLA class I total loss phenotype in this CRC soubgroup (Fernandez et al. 2000). Indeed, Cabrera et al. showed in 2003 that the transcriptional dowregulation of LMP7 and TAP2 genes were responsible for total loss of HLA-I expression in MSS-CRC group (Cabrera et al. 2003a). The involvement of TAP-1 downregulation in HLA-I loss in CRC have been also reported (Kaklamanis et al. 1994). Watson and coworkers published that immunosurveillance is active in colorectal cancer since downregulation but not complete loss of MHC class I expression correlates with a poor prognosis (Watson et al. 2006). These findings are probably related to the route used by CRC metastatic spread. Tumor cells with total loss of HLA class I supposedly will be destroyed by NK cells when travelling via the portal vein to the liver (Kloor et al. 2010).

A variety of colorectal carcinoma cell lines with different HLA-I altered expression have been reported: LS411 colorectal cell line shows a chromosomal breakpoint in the HLA-A11 allele (HLA allele loss, phenotype No. IV) (Browning et al. 1993b); C08, C012,and C067 tumor cell lines display concordant HLA altered phenotypes compatible with HLA haplotype loss (phenotype No.II) (Ramal et al. 2000b) and HLA A,B locus-specific downregulation (phenotype No. III) (Smith et al. 1988; Lopez-Nevot et al. 1989). A recent Epidemiological study carried out by a Colorectal Cancer Consortium (GECCO) at the National Cancer Institute (NCI) reported a genome-wide association study integrating data obtained from 592 cases (Grasso et al. 2018) plus 619 previously published primary tumor cases (Giannakis et al. 2016). This study included 179 MSI-H hypermutated cases (around 15%) showing that these tumors frequently undergo immune escape throught MHC antigen presentation pathway alterations, including β2 microglobulin mutations. These results confirm previously published reports by different groups (Kloor et al. 2010; Bernal et al. 2012a, b) and add new information about the high frequency of mutations found in HLA A, B and C HLA individual class I genes.

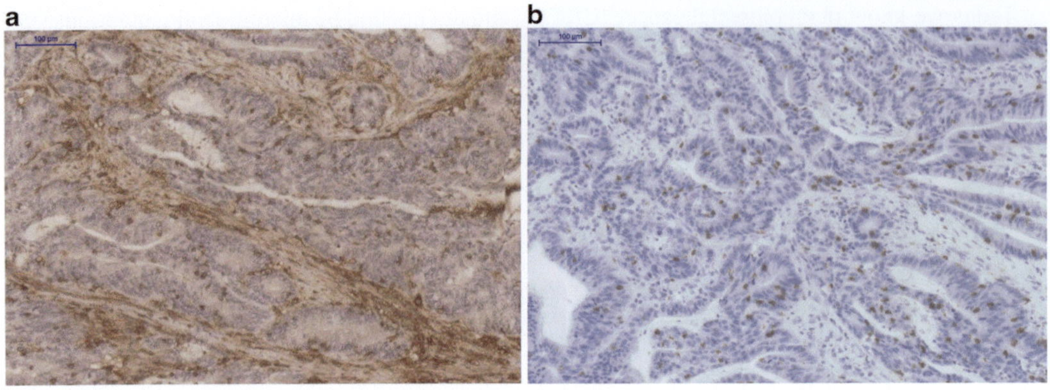

Fig. 2.15 **MSI-H Colorectal carcinoma.** (**a**) Tumor tissue is HLA-I negative (HC-10 MoAb) and is heavily infiltrated with CD8 positive T lymphocytes (**b**)

An interesting observation made in HLA class I negative MSI-H colorectal carcinomas is that they are heavily infiltrated by lymphocytes (Buckowitz et al. 2005; Bernal et al. 2012b). According to the data obtained in lung, melanomas, bladder etc. (Aptsiauri et al. 2018), in HLA negative tumor lymphocytes should be located outside the tumor nest, in the surrounding stroma. However in MSI-H HLA class I negative colorectal cancer, lymphocytes are masively infiltrating the tumor niche. The reason is yet unknown with several open possibilities "on the table" (Kloor et al. 2010). See Fig. 2.15.

Endometrial Cancer

Endometrial cancer can be divided in two types: Type I consist of endometroid carcinomas and type II are clear cell and serous papillary carcinomas. In type I tumors microsatellite instability (MSI) is a frequent fenomenon with the incidences around 20–30% as compared to 0–10% detected in type II cancer (Karamurzin and Rutgers 2009). MSI is caused by a failure of the mismatch repair (MMR) system to cut out and replace the mismatching DNA strains. MMR deficiency leads to the accumulation of single based-pair mismatches as well as small insertions and deletions in tandem repeats known as microsatellites. A similar phenomenon happens in a subset of colorectal carcinomas i.e. the MSI-H group (Ionov et al. 1993; Kloor et al. 2010). Tissue microarrays containing epithelial endometrial carcinoma tissue from 554 patients were stained for HLA class I heavy chain and β2 microglobulin. MHC-I downregulation in neoplastic cells was observed in 48% of cases and was a predictor of worse survival (Bijen et al. 2010). In a selected cohort of 486 endometrial cancers patients, HLA class I antigens and Mismacht repair proteins (MMR) were investigated together by immunohistochemistry. Loss of HLA B/C expression was found in 37% of cases in the group of endometroid with MMR protein loss compared to 25% in the MMR positive group (De Jong et al. 2012) The molecular mechanisms responsible for HLA class I downregulation, including β2 microglobulin mutations, was not analyzed. The available information on HLA-I phenotypes in endometrial cancer comes from a single laboratory and will require in the future more detailed analysis.

Esophageal Carcinoma

In 1995 Rocket et al reported for the first time that esophageal carcinomas also lose HLA class I expression. As many as 65% of the cases had weak or no HLA class I expression (Rockett et al. 1995). Normal oesophageal tissue showed positive staining for HLA-ABC in the basal layers of the oesophageal squamous ephitelium and on the ephitelial cells of the submucosal glands. HLA DR was not detected in either of these cell types.

In another study Nie et al showed that 89% of esophageal tumor tissues display loss of HLA-A, B and C molecules whereas all normal epithelial tissues are stained intensely with w6/32 MoAb (Nie et al. 2001). The mechanism/s underlying these HLA-I losses seems to be diverse. HLA class I transcriptional inactivation caused by DNA hypermethylation seems to play an important role in this process as well as LOH for HLA A,B and C genes loci (Nie et al. 2001). The third report on HLA class I expression in esophageal carcinomas showed locus especific losses in HLA-A (59%), HLA-B (41%) and β2 microglobulin (35%) respectively, using 84 paraffin embedded tumor tissue samples (Yang et al. 2008). In the same report HLA-I losses in 49 fresh samples showed similar results. In the future it will be necessary to define the different molecular mechanisms that are responsible for HLA-class I losses in oesophageal cancer and to estimate the percentage of "irreversible/hard" versus "reversible/soft" molecular mechanisms.

Gastric Carcinoma

We reported in 1989 analysis of HLA expression in 30 cryopreserved primary gastric carcinomas, 27 autologous metastasis and 25 autologous gastric mucosa (Ferron et al. 1989; Lopez-Nevot et al. 1989). The results obtained showed a complete absence of HLA ABC antigens in 10% of the samples and a variable expression in two cases using monoclonal antibodies against HLA-I monomorphic determinants. Additional HLA-I losses were detected with anti HLA-B locus specific MoAbs (15%) and the final number of HLA-I losses increased up to 25%. The remaining 22 primary tumors presented a homogeneously positive HLA class I expression. When the autologous mucosa was analyzed only 12 out of 25 speciments were homogeneously stained suggesting that this normal tissue may lack HLA-I or have a very weak expression in a high proportion of cases. Indeed, the majority of studied gastric carcinomas presented a higher HLA-ABC expression than autologous mucosa. The HLA expression in gastric carcinomas and autologous mucosa resemble that observed in renal cell carcinomas where the expression in autologous mucosa is weaker than in the corresponding tumour tissue (Saenz-Lopez et al. 2010). However other studies have reported that the HLA-I expression is downregulated in gastric cancer as compared to the normal mucosa (Klein et al. 1991; Shen et al. 2005). Shen et al studied 185 paraffin embedded speciments of gastric cancer and 22 controls of normal gastric mucosa. They found the expression of HLA-B/C locus expression was negative or heterogeneous in 60–70% of the histological grade I, II and III tumors as compared with the gastric mucosa. Ishigami and coworkers studied paraffin embedded gastric tumors using MoAb EMR8-5 that recognizes a monomorphic HLA class I determinant and indicated than 80% of the patients had a positive expression of HLA class I and was higher in differentiated tumors. These authors also considered the possibility that the HLA expression in gastric cancer might be related to inflammation since normal mucosa is exposed to external estimulae (Ishigami et al. 2008). A recent study by Lee et al in 189 gastric cancer tissues using also the EMR8-5 MoAb showed that 55% of tumours had a strongly positive HLA-I expression, 40% were weak positive and 5% showed negative expression. The downregulation was not associated with patient prognosis (Lee et al. 2011). In the future more detailed HLA analysis is required using cryopreserved tissues and a broad panel of anti HLA-I MoAbs in order to accurately define the patterns of HLA-I expression and the molecular mechanisms of HLA-I losses in gastric carcinomas.

Glioblastoma

Glioblastoma is the most lethal adult primary brain tumor. The median life expectancy is 14 months. Effector T cell infiltration has been found to be associated with longer survival of patients (Yang et al. 2010; Lohr et al. 2011). Facoeti and coworkers using immunohistochemistry in paraphin embedded tumor tissues demonstrated that HLA class I expression is downregulated in approximately 50% of cases (Facoetti et al. 2005). An important molecular mechanism responsible for these HLA alterations is loss of heterozigocity (LOH) in chromosome 6 associated with HLA haplotype loss (Yeung et al. 2013). Forty one percent of glioblastoma patients presented LOH in the HLA-I region that was associated with shorter overall survival. Interestingly, HLA class I positive expression correlated with intratumoral but not perivascular CD8+ T cell infiltration (Yeung et al. 2013). It will be necessary in the future to define if other molecular mechanisms are responsible for HLA-I downregulation in glioblastoma.

Head and Neck Carcinoma

Head and neck cancer is the sixth most common form of cancer worldwide (Vokes et al. 1993). More than 90% of head and neck cancers are squamous cell carcinomas. The oral cavity is the most common site within the head and neck tumors and the larynx is the second one. Many histopathological criteria have been introduced as differentiation and prognostic parameters (Pera et al. 1986). Head and neck squamous cell carcinomas derive from HLA class-I positive epithelia. We reported in 1989 that benign (squamous metaplasic epithelium and squamous papilloma) and *in situ* carcinomas are HLA class I positive (Esteban et al. 1989; Garrido et al. 1993), but many HLA altered phenotypes can be found in invasive carcinomas (Garrido et al. 1997a) (Fig. 2.16). Mattijssen and coworkers compared the HLA expression in 66 paraffin embedded head and neck squamous cell carcinomas with the corresponding frozen sections of the lesions. A high percentaje of matching score was found between the reactivity of HC10 and w6/32 monoclonal antibodies (Mattijssen et al. 1991). A strong correlation between the degree of differentiation and class I antigen expression has been found in laryngeal carcinomas (Lopez-Nevot et al. 1989). HLA class I total loss and tumor aggressiveness have also been correlated in laryngeal carcinomas (Esteban et al. 1990). It have been suggested that the loss of expression of HLA class I alleles may have prognostic implications and loss of expression of one or more alleles at the HLA-A or B locus was observed in 50% of the primary tumors tested (Grandis et al. 2000). In summary, seventy-nine percent of laryngeal tumors present an HLA class I altered phenotype (Cabrera et al. 1997, 2000). The presence of tumor infiltrating lymphocytes (TILs) was analyzed in relation to HLA-I expression and long-term follow up in a series of sixty primary laryngeal carcinomas (Esteban et al. 1996). From these data, we conclude that neither complete loss of HLA class I molecules nor tumour infiltrating lymphocytes influence survival in squamous cell carcinoma of the larynx. In this study

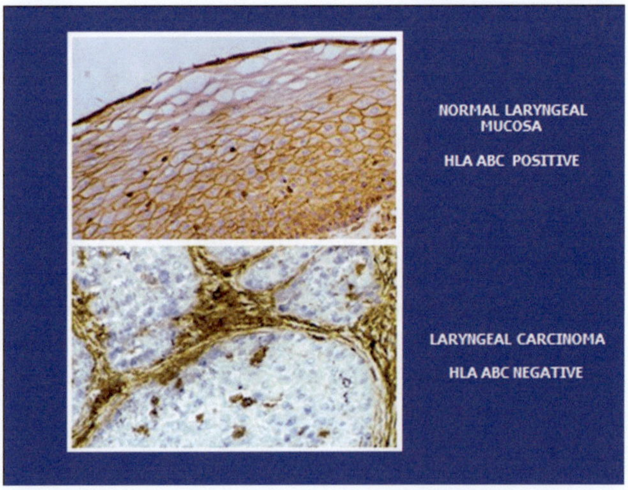

Fig. 2.16 **HLA class I antigen expression in a laryngeal mucosa and a laryngeal carcinoma**. The mucosa is HLA-I positive and the carcinoma is negative using the w6/32 MoAb that recognizes a common HLA A,B,C determinant

we did not distinguish between lymphocytes located inside the tumor nest and in the stroma.

Regarding the molecular basis of the defect in HLA class I expression in these tumors, we have reported that transcriptional regulation of HLA expression is likely to be involved (Esteban et al. 1989). It has been also published that downregulation of HLA class I expression in head and neck squamous cell carcinomas is correlated with loss of chromosomal region 6p21.3 (including the HLA complex) (Feenstra et al. 1999a). LOH for 6p21.3 is a frequent event occurring in 49% of the tumors with downregulated HLA class I expression. In addition, it has been reported by two independent groups that β2 microglobulin mutations are not involved in the generation of HLA class I total loss in laryngeal carcinomas (Feenstra et al. 1999b, 2000; Fernandez et al. 2000), but exists a high level of chromosome 15 aneuploidy (Koene et al. 2004). Defects in the HLA class I antigen processing machinery in head and neck squamous cell carcinoma have been also reported (Meissner et al. 2005; Ogino et al. 2006). Furthermore precise analysis of the molecular basis for HLA class I total or allelic lose in head and neck carcinomas are required. In this context the presence of HPV 16 sequences in laryngeal carcinomas has been demonstrated (Perez-Ayala et al. 1990) indicating that this oncogenic virus can be also directly involved in the downregulation of HLA class I molecules as it was demonstrated in cervical carcinoma (Bartholomew et al. 1997).

Hepatocellular Carcinoma

Hepatocelular carcinoma represent an "exception to the rule" because has increased HLA class I expression. Paterson and coworkers reported in 1988 the study of HLA class I and II in 70 samples of cryopreserved hepatocellular carcinoma (HCC) tissue samples (Paterson et al. 1988). In comparison with normal hepatocytes, the majority (94%) of HCC show higher levels of HLA ABC antigens. 45% of the speciments showed HLA-DR expression that was heterogeneously distributed. A weak membranous staining of HLA-DR was observed on normal hepatocytes with an intense staining within sinusoids (endothelial and Kupffer cells). It has been proposed that the promielocytic leukemia protooncogene (PML) controls the transcription of class I genes in HCC, because PML and HLA class I molecules were concordantly upregulated and this gene might be one of the mechanism that leads to the increased expression of class I in HCC (Xia et al. 2007). HLA expression was also studied in hepatocarcinoma cell lines. HLA-B and C molecules were not detected in six out of seven lines using flow cytometry analysis indicating that hepatocellular carcinoma cell lines lose or decrease B and C alleles (Kurokohchi et al. 1996). However, other reports show opposite results (Wadee et al. 1994; Matsui et al. 2002). Further studies are required to precisely define the HLA expression in hepatocellular carcinomas.

Lymphoma & Leukemia

HLA class I loss can be also observed in lymphoma and leukemia. A pioneer work was published by Massucci and coworkers (Massucci et al. 1987). They reported that Epstein-Bar virus induced Burkitt lymphoma has a selective downregulation of HLA-A11 alloespecificity and are resistant to lysis by the HLA-A11 restricted CTLs generated by stimulation with the autologous lymphoblastoid cell line. A report of an HLA analysis in 397 acute myeloid and 186 acute lymphoid leukemias using a complement dependent cytotoxicity assay detected downregulation in 2% of AML and ALL patients in complete remission and in 8–15% in the group with blasts (Brouwer et al. 2002). The HLA-I downregulation or complete loss were confirmed using flow cytometry. Interestingly, treatment of the cells with α or γ interferon could restore HLA class-I expression and T cell recognition. Another report took advantage of a large panel of anti HLA class I allele-especific human monoclonal antibodies produced and characterized by A. Mulder in Leiden. This analysis was performed at the HLA-I allelic level comparing the expression in leukemias with that of autologous normal cells (Demanet et al. 2004). Downregulation of HLA-A and/or B alloespecificities was present in the majority of the patients studied. Interestingly, the downregulation affects HLA alleles of the HLA-Bw6 soubgroup, which does not interact with NK cell receptors. These results suggest that the selective down-regulation of HLA-A and HLA-Bw6 specificities and the preservation of HLA-Bw4 provide leukemic cells with a combined escape mechanism from T lymphocytes and from NK cells (Demanet et al. 2004). A group of 20 B-CLL, 16 B-ALL and 19 AML were studied using the same panel of human monoclonal antibodies (Verheyden et al. 2009). This study showed a marked reduction of cell surface expression of HLA-C alleles. Taken together the published data on HLA-I expression in leukemia it seems that tumor cells in this malignancy use altered HLA-I phenotypes to escape both T and NK cells responses. It also provides evidences that NK cells can survey and kill HLA-I deficient leukemic cells due to the the absence of an NK inhibitory signal provided by the complementary HLA-I molecule. These data strongly suggest that the biallelic system Bw4/Bw6 described by JJ van Rood in his doctoral thesis in 1964 could be playing a major role in the NK escape route used by leukemias (Verheyden et al. 2009).

A clear example of T cells involvement in the rejection of haploidentical haematopoyetic stem cell transplantation in leukemias has been reported (Vago et al. 2009; Villalobos et al. 2010). Leukemic cells can escape from donor antileukemic T cells through the loss of the mismatched HLA haplotype. The HLA haplotype that differ from the donor´s haplotype has been lost because of adquired uniparental disomy at chromosome 6p. This event leads to leukemia relapse (Vago et al. 2012). Despite these examples of leukemic relapse happen after an alloimmune interaction, the mechanism of escape is again the LOH of the missmached HLA haplotype. The data summarizes here on HLA class I losses in leukemias point to the involvement of T cells reacting against tumor antigens presented by HLA- I molecules and the generation of the escape variant with the loss of the HLA restriction element. Later, NK cells take the lead and can kill the HLA B and C deficient cells in the blood but again HLA Bw4 positive leukemic variants appear that can escape NK cell responses (Demanet et al. 2004). It is becaming evident that NK cell could play a major role in killing circulating tumor cells of heamatological origin similarly to the colorectal cancer cells disseminating via blood circulation to liver via the portal vein (Kloor et al. 2010). In this context, we observed the aberrant expression of HLA-E in leukemia-derived cell lines. HLA-E is a non classical HLA-I molecule that interact with NK inhibitory receptor CD94NKG2A,D and therefore is capable of inhibit the NK cell killing promoting an additional tumour escape mechanism (Marin et al. 2003). An interesting observation has been recently published by Dr Ruiz-Cabello and his team in my lab. Low-risk myelodysplatic syndrome with low mutational rate can have a poor prognosis if an HLA haplotype loss occurs during transformation to acute myeloid leukemia (Montes et al. 2018). These data reinforce the idea that leukemias are also under control of T and NK cell immunesurveillance.

In contrast to leukemias, lymphomas are considered as solid tumors since they grow inside the lymph nodes. They derive from malignant transformation of T and B lymphocytes. HLA class I losses were described also in B cell lymphomas long time ago (Moller et al. 1987) and were associated with an aggressive clinical behavior (Amiot et al. 1998). Loss of heterozygocity is a frequent but not exclusive mechanism for HLA dowregulation in non-Hodking lymphomas. LOH was detected in 9 out of 14 cases. HLA class I losses were described in 5 out of 15 cases in addition to HLA-A and B locus downregulation (Drenou et al. 2004). β2 microglobulin aberrations were reported in diffuse large B cell lymphoma (DLBCL) of the testis and the central nervous system (Jordanova et al. 2003). A recent report in DLBCL showed HLA class I total loss detected in more than 60%, also with the involvement of β2 microglobulin mutations (Challa-Malladi et al. 2011).

Lung Carcinoma

The expression of HLA antigens in lung carcinoma has been extensively estudied with a general consensus that HLA class I loss is a frequent aberration in this type of malignancy (Garrido et al. 2018). Carcinoma of the lung is the most common cancer in males. The subdivision of bronchogenic carcinoma into different clinicopathological entities, such as small cell carcinoma of aggressive behavior and non-small cell carcinoma of slower evolution is well established and used in the clinic. The available evidence suggests that all the major subtypes of bronchogenic carcinoma arise from the basal cells of the bronchial epithelium, which has endodermal origin. During the early phases of neoplastic development the malignant cells tend to differentiate as squamous cells, glandular cells, large undifferentiated epithelial cells, or small cells.The prognosis in patients with lung cancer is determined by several factors, the most important of which are the specific histological diagnosis, tumor stage and host performance status (Carbone 1997).

Normal lung tissue (pneumocytes and epithelial respiratory cells) expresses HLA class I antigens (Redondo et al. 1991a, b; Garrido et al. 1993). However, HLA class I antigen expression is frequently modified in lung tumors. We have shown that the loss of HLA class I antigen in lung cancer bears a significant relationship with two markers of biological aggressiveness: the degree of tumor cell differentiation and the presence of aneuploidy (Redondo et al. 1991a, 1997). HLA class I total loss is the most frequent phenotype in this type of tumor. The loss of HLA-A, B, and C molecules was found in 38% of all lung tumors and is usually accompanied by loss of β2 microglobulin. Selective loss of A and B locus has also been found in bronchogenic carcinomas (Redondo et al. 1991a; Korkolopoulou et al. 1996). The available data indicate a frequency of 8% for selective HLA-A locus loss, although this percentage would probably be higher in a more thorough analysis. This was implied by a study of HLA class I allelic loss. In a series of 93 specimens of non-small cell lung carcinomas, HLA-A2 allele was lost in 27% of the cases (Korkolopoulou et al. 1996). The molecular mechanisms for these alterations have not been fully elucidated, but data from different laboratories suggest that mutations in the β2 microglobulin gene (Chen et al. 1996a) and in TAP1 (Chen et al. 1996b) are mechanisms responsible for HLA alterations, as is the case for lung carcinoma cell lines H2009 and H1436, respectively. Loss of TAP1 is also involved in the abnormal HLA class I expression in other lung carcinoma tissues and cell lines (Korkolopoulou et al. 1996; Singal et al. 1998; Lou et al. 2005). HLA haplotype loss is also an important mechanism in lung cancer leading to irreversible/hard altered HLA phenotypes as seen in a large variety of tumors (So et al. 2005; Perea et al. 2017).

We have recently analyzed the HLA-I expression in a series of 57 tumor tissues from patients with lung carcinomas in correlation with immune cell infiltration (Perea et al. 2017). We found that 49% of lung carcinomas were completely negative for HLA-I and 5% showed a selective HLA-A downregulation. In 48% we detected a positive expression but with a percentage of HLA-I negative cells between 10% and 25%. The HLA negative phenotype was produced by a combination of HLA haplotype loss and a transcriptional downregulation of β2 microglobulin and LMP2 and LMP7 antigen presentation machinery genes. We also obtained data demonstrating that HLA-I loss caused by β2 microglobulin mutations is not very common in NSCLC. However, LOH in chromosome 6 seems to have highly relevance as a mechanism of HLA-I loss in NSCLC as we have recently shown (Perea et al. 2017). Similar data was reported by McGranahan and co-authors (MacGranahan et al. 2017).

The analysis and localization of different immune cell populations in lung cancer tissue revealed the presence of two main patterns (See Figs. 2.17a and 2.17b). One pattern is characterized by a positive HLA-I expression and intratumoral infiltration with CD8+ T cells and M1 macrophages. We named it as "immune permissive phase ". The other pattern demonstrates negative HLA-I expression in tumour cells with CD8+ T cells restrained outside the tumour nest in the

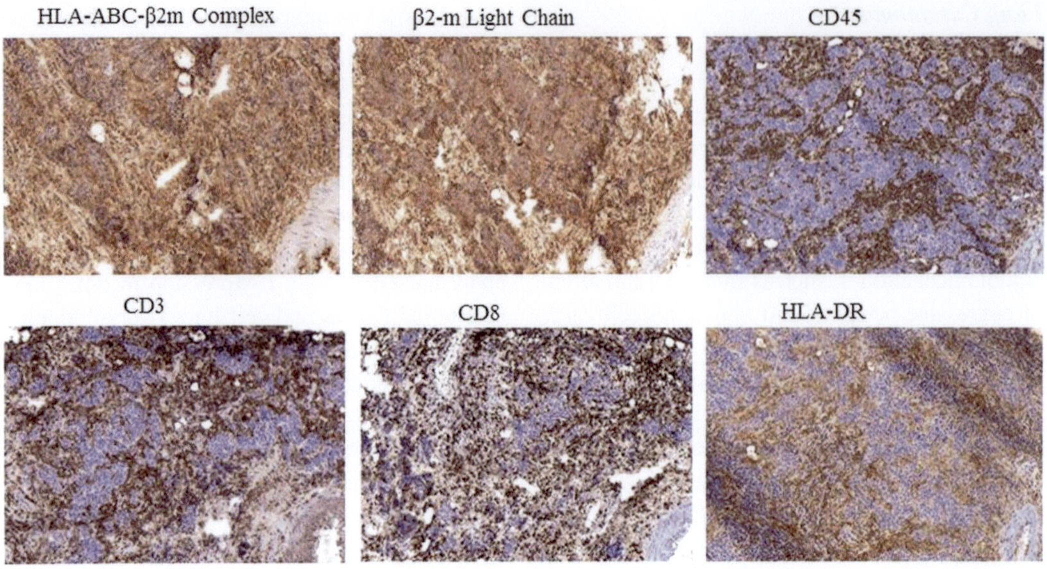

Fig. 2.17a Tissue architecture in HLA class I positive tumors. Tumor tissues obtained from a patient diagnosed with non-small cell lung cancer (NSCLC) were immunostained with monoclonal antibodies against HLA-class-I, β2-microglobulin, HLA class-II, CD8, CD3, and CD45 molecules. Most of the cancer cells are HLA-I positive and tumors are heavily infiltrated with CD8+ T cells. The tissue structure is "permissive", allowing TILs to enter the tumor mass and get into a direct contact with cancer cells. Tumor parenquima and stroma cannot be distinguished when staining for HLA-I. This pattern in HLA-I positive tumors is different from that observed in HLA-I negative tissues described in Fig. 2.17b (see below). (Reprinted by permission of MDPI: Vaccines (Basel) Garrido et al. 2017)

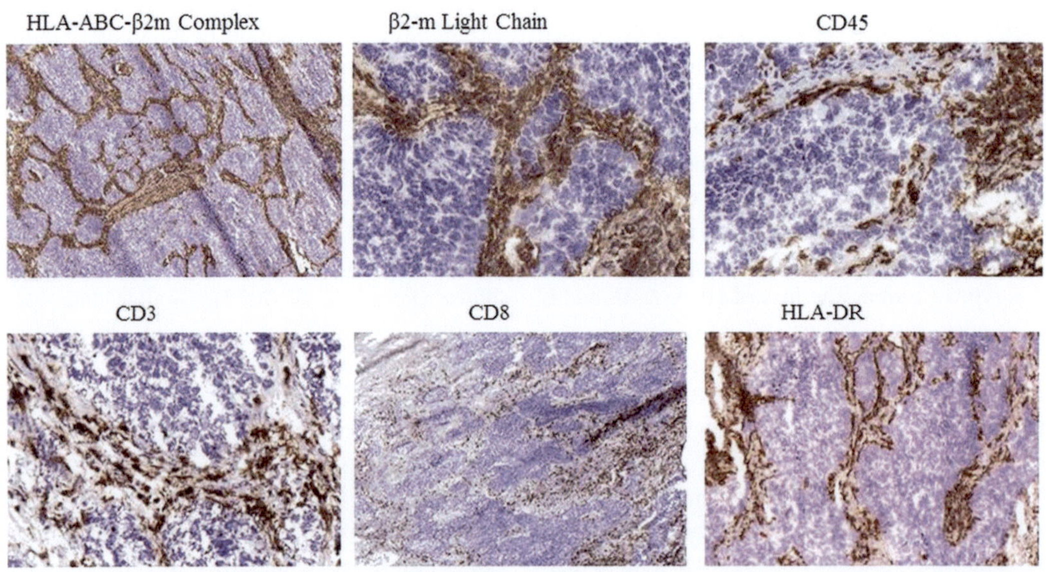

Fig. 2.17b Tissue architecture in HLA class I negative tumors. A lung cancer tumor tissue from another patient is negative for both HLA class-I and II. T cells and other leukocytes are restricted exclusively to the peri-tumoral stroma that surrounds the tumor nest in a "non-permissive" tissue structure. Tumor tissue is composed only of HLA-I negative tumor cells. There is a clear separation between tumor parenquima and stroma. Tumor nodes are composed exclusively of tumor cells without any infiltrating cell. (Reprinted by permission of MDPI: Vaccines (Basel) Garrido et al. 2017)

stroma surrounding the tumor niche: "an encapsulated phase" (Garrido et al. 2017). These data strongly suggest that the transition from HLA-I positive expression to HLA class I loss is associated with the decrease in tumor infiltration with T cells and with a significant tissue structure reorganization (see Fig. 2.10a–c). Furthermore, when we analized the density and composition of tumor T cell infiltration in non-small lung cell carcinoma in relation to PD-L1 and HLA-I expression we found that positive HLA-I expression is independent of PD-L1 status and HLA expression is the key factor determining the increased density of the immune infiltrate (Perea et al. 2018).

Melanoma

Melanoma has always attracted the interest of immunologist because of the observation of frequent mononuclear cell infiltration associated with spontaneous regressions (Cochran et al. 1988) and is one of the few tumours responding to immunotherapy. Melanoma is the least common cancer among the main types of skin cancer (basal cell carcinoma and squamous cell carcinoma), but it accounts for three-fourths of all deaths from skin cancer. Currently, it is the most rapidly increasing form of cancer, and recent statistics have shown a doubling in the number of new cases during the past 15 years. The most important risk factor that has been identified is exposure to sunlight, especially during childhood. There are two distinct phases of growth in malignant melanoma. During the first noninvasive phase the neoplastic cells spread horizontally without breaking the basal membrane. This phase may last 2–5 years. The second phase is characterized by rapid vertical growth, leading to the invasion of the dermis. Clark's levels establish the degree of dermal invasion in melanoma and Breslow's thickness quantifies the local growth of the tumor (Clark et al. 1969; Breslow 1975).

It has been proposed that many immunological events are involved in the pathogenesis of malignant melanoma and that abnormalities in HLA class I antigen expression by melanoma cells may have adverse effects on the clinical course of the disease. HLA studies in melanoma were performed in a pioneer work by Pellegrino and coworkers. Melanoma was the first human tumour in which HLA class I losses were identified by several groups (Pellegrino et al. 1977; Winchester et al. 1978; Wilson et al. 1979). Melanoma was also the first human tumor in which a specific antigen presented by MHC class I molecules and recognized by T lymphocytes was identified (MAGE) (Van der Bruggen et al. 1991). These genes encode proteins that contribute a peptide tumor antigen presented by the HLA products to cytotoxic T lymphocytes.

HLA class I antigen expression has been demonstrated in normal melanocytes by electron microscopy (Van Duinen et al. 1984). The reports of Dirk Ruiter and coworkers have shown that benign nevi are class I negative, whereas dysplastic nevi are class I positive (Ruiter et al. 1982, 1991). HLA class I losses in malignant melanoma have been shown in many tumor samples both metastastic tissues and cultured tumor cell lines. Most of the initial studies of HLA and melanoma were done with mAbs that recognized nonpolymorphic determinants of the HLA-A, -B, and -C molecules. The differences observed in the data reported (Turbitt and Mackie 1981; Ruiter et al. 1982; D'Alessandro et al. 1987; Lopez-Nevot et al. 1986; Holzmann et al. 1987; Ernstoff et al. 1985) can be explained by the different sensitivities of the immunohistochemical staining procedures used, the different nature of the lesions tested, differences in antibody specificities, and differences in the criteria used to define a positive or negative lesion. In these studies HLA class I losses were observed in both primary and metastatic lesions (Holzmann et al. 1987). The phenotypic alterations were related to histopathological malignancy criteria and tumor progression (Lopez-Nevot et al. 1988; Ruiter et al. 1991). Using a large battery of mAbs (locus or allele specific), which define HLA losses more accurately, studies of melanoma tumors have shown that approximately 63% of primary melanoma lesions present HLA phenotypic alterations (Marincola et al. 1994; Garrido et al. 1997b). In this context, a high frequency of allele specific downregulation of HLA class I expression has been reported in uveal melanoma cell lines (Hurks et al. 2000).

Several molecular mechanisms underlie the HLA phenotypes found in melanoma tumors. The most common molecular alteration responsible for total HLA class I loss in melanoma cells is a mutation in the β2 microglobulin gene, which results in loss of functional β2 microglobulin expression (Natali et al. 1989; D'Urso et al. 1991; Wang et al. 1993; Hicklin et al. 1998). Our laboratory described β2 microglobulin mutations in a melanoma tumor cell line (GR34) (Perez et al. 1999) and in two melanoma lines of patients immunized with MAGE peptides (BB74-MEL and LB1622-MEL) (Benitez et al. 1998; Lopez-Nevot et al. 2002) (see Fig. 2.18). These mutations are the reason why the tumors of both patients progressed despite peptide immunotherapy. Loss of heterozigocity at 6p21 has been described as one of the most frequent karyotypic abnormalities that appear in human malignant melanoma (Real et al. 1998; Mendez et al. 2001). We identified a new HLA class I altered phenotype that is the result of a combination of HLA-B and C locus downregulation and HLA haplotype loss. The alteration was found in two melanoma cell lines generated from two patients; one derived from an *in vivo* lesion (FM37 cell line) and the other was obtained after *in vitro* immunoselection (R22.2 cell line) (Real et al. 1998). The final result was a melanoma tumor cell that expressed a single HLA class I allele. A transcriptional suppression of HLA-B locus specific products in melanoma was described to be associated with c-myc oncogene activation (Peltenburg and Schrier 1994). An example that adds further complexity to the pattern of HLA altered phenotypes in melanoma tumors is represented by human melanoma cell line FO-1 (Martayan et al. 1999). A minimum of three defects hinder class I expression in FO-1 cells: the lack of β2 microglobulin, a low expression of TAP, and poor HLA class I-calreticulin interaction. A structural alteration in two distinc components of the antigen presentation machinery was also reported in melanomas (Seliger et al.

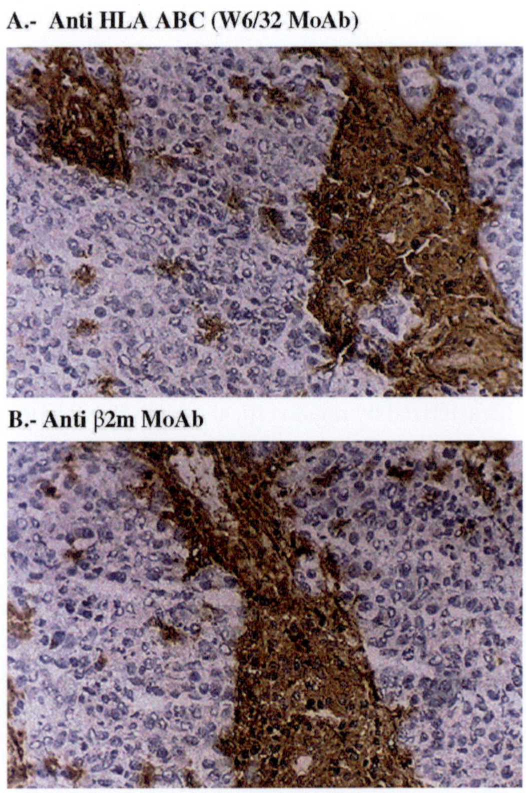

Fig. 2.18 HLA class I loss in a melanoma metastatic tumor tissue. This patient was immunized with MAGE1-HLA-A1 peptide at the Ludwig Institute in Brussels and did not respond to therapy. We showed that the tissue was HLA-I negative due to a β2 microglobulin gene mutation and LOH in chromosome 15th (see Benitez et al. 1998). (Reprinted by permission of Wiley: Benitez et al. 1998)

2001). All these defects can impair normal cell surface recognition by cytotoxic T cells (Hicklin et al. 1999)

All the altered HLA class I phenotypes described in this book have been identified in melanoma tissues and melanoma cell lines (Real et al. 1998; Benitez et al. 1998; Mendez et al. 2008). In cooperation with Gustav Gaudernak in the Radium hospital in Oslo, we have recently followed the HLA expression in a primary melanoma lesion and autologous metastasis (del Campo et al. 2014). We found that the primary tumor was heterogeneous with positive and negative areas for HLA class I expression. Using a laser capture microdissection technique we analyzed a HLA-I negative area and found a point mutation in the β2 microglobulin gene. Interestingly, the same point mutation in the same codon was found in an homogeneous HLA-I negative autologous subcutaneous metastasis produced 16 month later (del Campo et al. 2014). These data strongly suggest an active ongoing T cell mediated immuneselection of HLA-I negative variants.

Neuroblastoma

Neuroblastoma, a tumor of neuroectodermal origin, is one of the most common solid extracranial tumor in childhood with a poor survival rate. At early stages it usually undergoes spontaneous regression and has an excellent prognosis, however at stage 4 tumours remain mostly resistance to therapy and correlate with poor prognosis with an overall survival of 45% (Berthold et al. 2003). It has been demonstrated that neuroblastoma expresses several cancer "germline" antigens such as those of the MAGE family and therefore might be a candidate for vaccination trials (Corrias et al. 1996; Soling et al. 1999). In vitro data are controversial regarding the susceptibility of neuroblastoma to T cell mediated lysis which might be explained by differences in the characteristic of the cell lines and the avidity of the CTLs used (Main et al. 1988; Sarkar and Nuchtern 2000). Another possible explanation is the absence or weak expression of the T cell restriction element, namely the MHC molecules. Lack of HLA class I antigens was demonstrated in human neuroblastoma cells in relation with TAP and tapasin expression (Corrias et al. 2001). In cooperation with the Memorial Sloan-Kettering Cancer Center (NY), the Fred Hutchinson Cancer center in Seattle and the Children Hospital in Cologne (Germany) we analyzed the HLA class I expression in seventeen cryopreserved neuroblastoma tissues using a broad panel of anti HLA class I and class II monoclonal antibodies as previously described (Cabrera et al. 2003b). None of the 17 tumours was positive with any of the antibodies used for HLA-I and II (Wölf et al. 2005). Our results clearly show that neuroblastoma is an HLA class I and II negative tumor. In this context, early work on neuroblastoma showed an inverse correlation between MHC class I expression and amplification or overexpression of the N-myc proto-oncogene (Bernards et al. 1986; Van't Veer et al. 1993; Cheng et al. 1996). Neuroblastoma cell lines and primary tumor speciments revealed a low or undetectable expression of MHC class I and II molecules but inducible by IFN-γ (Lampson et al. 1985; Whelan et al. 1985). Since neuroblastoma tumors derive from cells of neuroectodermal origin that are most probably MHC class I negative (Daar et al. 1984), the absence of HLA class I in these tumors cannot be considered as a "loss". Encouraging results of antigen specific immunity in neuroblastoma patient mediated by T cell recognition of NY-ESO-1 especific killing (Rodolfo et al. 2003) clearly indicate that further investigation on neuroblastoma is needed to see if T cell mediated immunotherapy can be successfully proposed in this tumor considering that HLA class I and II antigens can be upregulated as demonstrated by different authors (Sugimoto et al. 1989).

Ovarian Cancer

In 2002 Le and coworkers reported the study of HLA class I expression in ovarian carcinoma (Le et al. 2002). Later Vitale et al. studied fifty-one formalin-fixed paraffin embedded primary ovarian carcinoma lesions using antibodies that recognize HLA-I monomorphic determinants and β2 microglobulin able to work in fixed tissues (Vitale et al. 2005). The results obtained showed an average of 37% of HLA-I losses. Few years later, Han et al. published the HLA-I analysis in a series of 150 invasive ovarian carcinomas using a similar approach. The majority of tumor samples had heterogeneous or positive staining and 35% had a clear HLA-I negative expression. Interestingly 58% of the samples were negative for Tapasin expression. The analysis of tumour infiltrating T cells revealed that the majority of the patients sowed some degree of intratumoral and peritumoral T cell infiltration suggesting that TILs may be a marker of antitumour response mechanism (Han et al. 2008). The molecular mechanisms underlying the HLA class I losses observed in ovarian carcinoma remain to be elucidated.

Pancreas Carcinoma

Cancer of the exocrine pancreas has a very poor prognosis in humans due to its difficulty in the diagnosis, late detection and the lack of effective therapy. There are few studies analyzing the expression of HLA antigens in pancreas cancer tissue. Our group reported that altered MHC class I expression is frequent in pancreas cancer (Torres et al. 1996). Using a combination of immunohistochemical, biochemical, and recombinant DNA approaches, we determined the prevalence and molecular basis of altered HLA class I expression in 26 pancreatic adenocarcinomas and 6 autologous tumor derived cell lines. The frequency of HLA class I losses according to analyses with monomorphic and locus-specific antibodies was 40%. The results obtained in one solid tumor tissue and its corresponding pancreatic tumor cell line (IMIM-PC2) indicate that LOH was responsible for the selective loss of MHC class I alleles in this tumor (Torres et al. 1996). Loss of heterocigosity (LOH) in chromosome 6 in pancreas cancer have been demonstrated in a series of pancreas tumour tissues (Ryschich et al. 2004).

A similar study found that the loss of HLA class I in pancreatic adenocarcinoma was in the range of 25% using antibodies against HLA-I monomorphic determinants (Scupoly et al. 1996). Recently, a study of HLA-I and tumor infiltrating lymphocytes in a series of pancreas tumour tissues showed a strong correlation between the number of TILs and the expression of HLA-I in the tumor nest, namely more HLA-I expression/more TILs and viceversa. These data strongly suggest that T lymphocytes are playing a major role in tumor destruction that produces a tumor composed only by HLA class I negative cells (Ryschich et al. 2005). In this study 46 primary tumors and 14 metastasis were analyzed. These authors showed that HLA class I total loss was detected in 30% and HLA A,B locus specific loss in 61% of cases. Metastasis showed a significant higher loss of monomorphic and locus-specific epitopes. The prognostic impact of HLA-I loss in pancreatic cancer have been also reported (Imai et al. 2017). This group analyzed the expression of PDL-1 and HLA class I in 36 pancreatic carcinomas by immunohistochemistry. PDL-1 expression correlated with tumour infiltration by $CD68^+$ and $FoxP3^+$ cells. PDL-1 negative and HLA class I positive high-expressing pancreas cancer tissues was significantly associated with higher numbers of infiltrating $CD8^+$ T cells. Low HLA class I expression was the only risk factor for poor survival. As indicated previously, HLA class I loss also occurs frequently in pancreas cancer but further studies are required to identify the molecular mechanism/s responsible in addition to loss of heterozigocity already described by Torres et al in 1996.

Prostate Carcinoma

HLA class I expression have been extensively analyzed by different groups in prostate cancer reporting that HLA-I losses are frequently found (Levin et al. 1994; Blades et al. 1995; Natali et al. 1989; Carretero et al. 2016). One of the factors that may influence prostate cancer progression is the expression of human leukocyte antigens in tumor cells. Prostate cancer is the second most common cause of death in most developed countries. In fact, about 80% of all cases occur in men who are 65 years of age or older. The Gleason score remains the best available prognostic factor for prostate cancer (Gleason and Mellinger 1974). HLA class I and II expression have been studied in benign prostatic hyperplasia, prostatic adenocarcinoma and metastatic prostate disease to define the extent of altered HLA expression and to determine whether HLA expression is related to disease progression (Blades et al. 1995; Garrido et al. 1997a; Lu et al. 2000) (see Fig. 2.19). These studies used mAbs which recognized both monomorphic determinants and HLA allelic products. In contrast to the HLA class I expression in the normal tissue and benign hyperplasias (Sharpe et al. 1994; Bander et al. 1997; Carretero et al. 2016), complete loss of HLA class I expression was observed in 34% of primary prostate cancers and 80% of lymph node metastases (Blades et al. 1995). Other authors estimated the frequency of HLA allelic loss (HLA-A2) in primary prostate cancer to be 51% (Natali et al. 1989). When individual allelic expression was assessed in combination with total loss, the minimum estimate of downregulation was 85% in the primary prostate cancer and 100% in the metastases. The concordant downregulation of proto-oncogene PML and major histocompatibility antigen HLA class I expression was described in high-grade prostate cancer (Zhang et al. 2003).

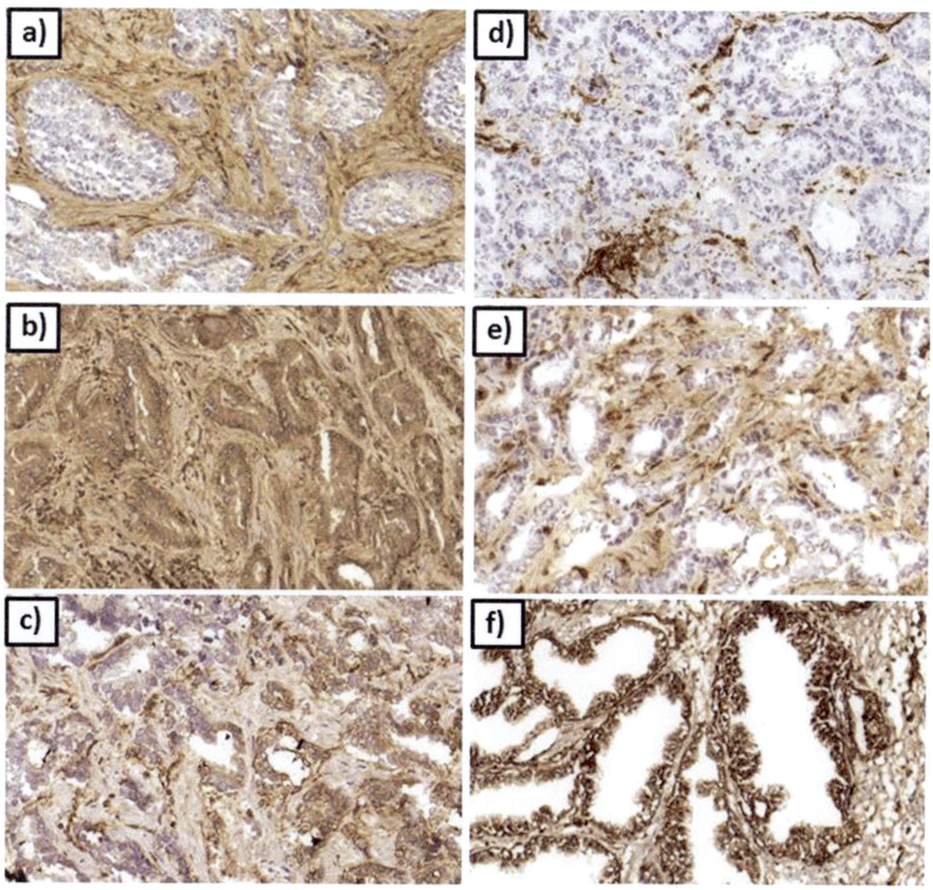

Fig. 2.19 Representative immunohistochemistry images of HLA class I expression in cryopreserved bening prostate hyperplasia and prostate cancer. HLA class I negative (**a**), positive (**b**) and heterogeneous expression (**c**). HLA A locus loss (**d**), HLA B locus heterogeneous loss (**e**) in prostate cancer. Positive expression in bening hyperplasia (**f**). (Reprinted by permission of Springer: Carretero et al. 2016)

Some tumor cell lines have been used in the search for the mechanisms that underlie these alterations of MHC class I expression in prostate tumors. We described that a nucleotide insertion in exon 4 is responsible for the absence of expression of an HLA-A*0301 allele in a prostate carcinoma cell line (Jimenez et al. 2001). The metastasis-derived cell line PPC-1 shows a regulatory defect in the antigen transport machinery that leads to specific underexpression of the TAP-2 gene product (Sanda et al. 1995). The analysis of 12 prostate cell lines derived from neoplastic tissue revealed different types of HLA-I alterations ranging from locus and allelic downregulation to a total absence of HLA-I expression (Carretero et al. 2016). We have recently reported that the percentage of HLA class I losses in prostate cancer tissue is 88%, including HLA total loss (50%), HLA A,B locus loss (26%) and HLA allelic loss (12%). Loss of heterozygosity at chromosome 6 including the HLA region was detected in 32% of the estudied tumors. Molecular analysis revealed a reduced expression of β2 microglobulin, TAP2, tapasin and NLRC5 mRNA in microdisected HLA-I negative tumors (Carretero et al. 2016). The study of HLA changes in tumor tissue of patients undergoing prostate immunotherapy is no doubt an open research field for future studies.

Renal Cell Carcinoma

The data reported on HLA-I expression in Renal Cell Carcinoma (RCC) suggest that this type of cancer is probably using a mechanisms other than HLA-I downregulation to escape T cell responses. Cordon-Cardo reported in 1991 that fresh-frozen tissue especiments of primary renal cell carcinomas showed dense HLA-I membrane immunohistological staining and 38% of the tumor samples showed a mixed pattern with positive and negative tumor cells (Cordon-Cardo et al. 1991). In the study reported by Buzello and Ackerman in 1994 studying 43 normal renal tissues and 48 primary RCC they found a strong expression of HLA-I in 40 samples and a homogeneous staining of all normal renal tissues (Buszello and Ackermann 1994). Kitamura et al published in 2007 that HLA-I was downregulated in 37.8% of clear cell renal carcinomas with no correlation with clinicopathological parameters (TNM, tumor size…etc) (Kitamura et al. 2007). Other reports in paraffin-embedded tumors revealed that "in contrast to other tumors, the study revealed an increase in HLA-ABC expression regardless of histological types and a more pronounced HLA class I staining was always observed in tumor cells as compared with normal adjacent tubule cells". In this study total HLA class-I loss was never observed (Cherif et al. 2003). In this context, we have obtained similar results in a series of 93 cryopreserved RCC and 31 normal renal tissue (Saenz-Lopez et al. 2010). In our study, HLA I expression was much higher on RCC cells than on normal renal tubular cells (see Fig. 2.20a, b). These findings were confirmed by a molecular analysis of HLA heavy chain and β2 microglobulin transcription levels using quantitative real-time polymerase chain reaction (PCR) on microdissected tissue samples of isolates tumor nest and autologous normal renal tubulae. There are also two independent findings that confirm this concept:HLA haplotype loss in RCC is a rare event (Maleno et al. 2004a) and numerous HLA-I and II binding peptides have been identified in RCC samples indicating a high expression of MHC molecules by renal tumors (Kruger et al. 2005; Dengjel et al. 2006). We have obtained data of high levels of proinflamatory cytokines associated with high levels of HLA-I in RCC tumor cells suggesting that may be involved in the upregulation of HLA expression during tumor progression (Romero et al. 2006). The low frequency of HLA-I loss in RCC can also explain why this cancer type has a high reponse rate to immunotherapy as it has been reported in different clinical trials using IL2 (Michael and Pandha 2003; Motzer et al. 1996; Marincola et al. 1995).

Thyroid Carcinoma

One recent study have showed that MHC class I expression was reduced or absent in 76% of papillary thyroid cancer and this HLA-I downregula-

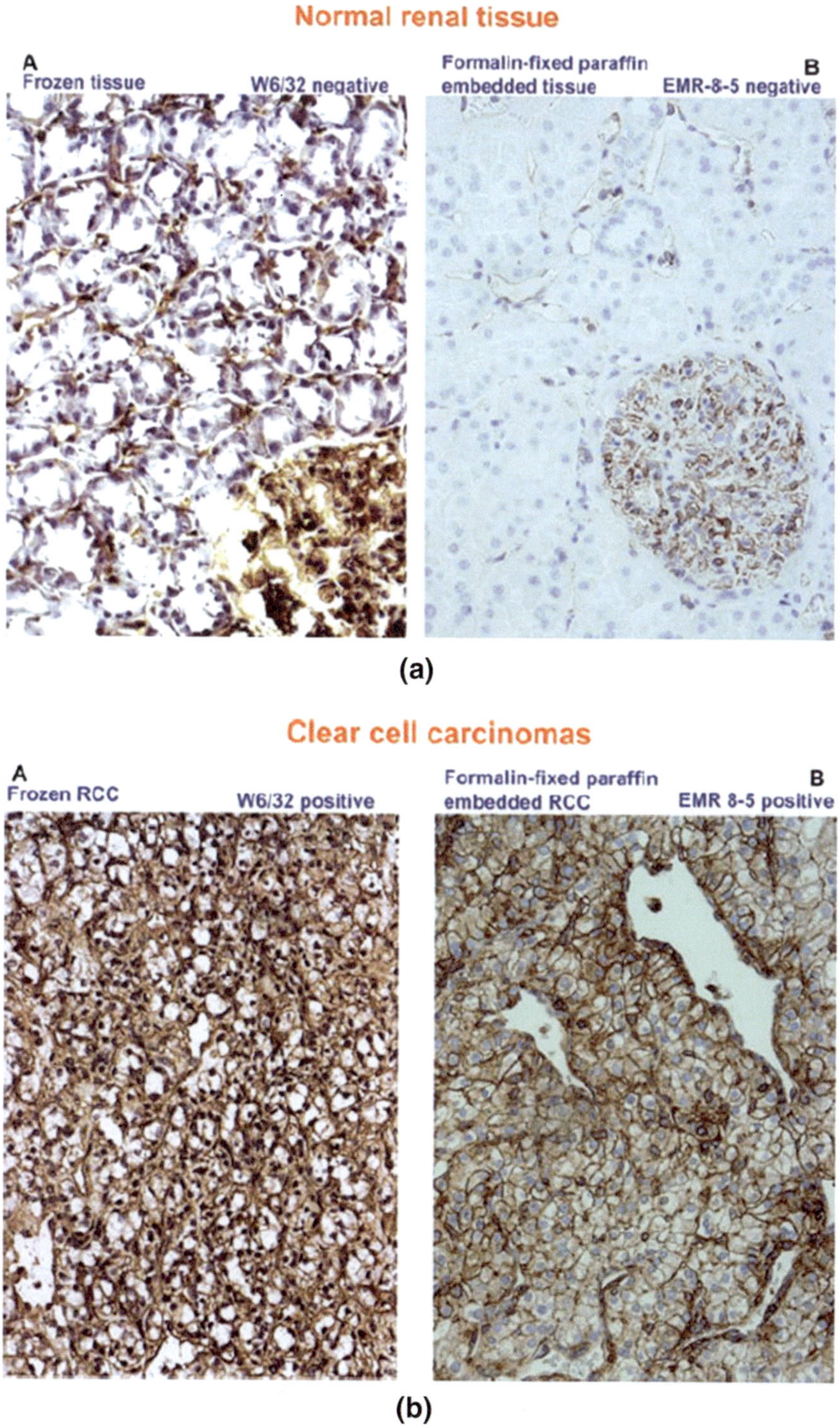

Fig. 2.20 HLA class-I expression in normal renal tissue and renal cell carcinoma. (**a**) Absence or weak expression on HLA-I antigens in cryopreserved and paraffin embedded normal renal tissues. (**b**) Positive staining of HLA class I antigens in clear cell carcinoma in cryopreserved and in paraffin embedded tissues. (Reprinted by permission of Wiley: Saenz-Lopez et al. 2010)

tion was associated with a decrease in tumor infiltrating lymphocytes (Angell et al. 2014). This type of cancer represents 90% of all thyroid malignancies.This study also indicate that a kinase inhibitor (Selumetinib) and IFN can induce HLA-I expression in thyroid cancer cell lines suggesting a "reversible/soft" mechanism present in this type of cancer. These findings are so far the only published results on HLA-I expression in thyroid tumors and confirm the idea that HLA-I deficient tumors are selected by TILs that are responsible for the killing of HLA-I positive tumor cells. The transition of HLA-I positive to HLA-I negative primary tumors we have proposed as a most likely chain of events also in thyroid tumors (Aptsiauri et al. 2018).

Uveal Melanoma

Loss of HLA A, B and C molecules (total, locus or allele loss) has been demonstrated in uveal melanoma by different authors (Jager et al. 2002). Ericsson and co-authors detected downregulation of HLA class I and β2 microglobulin expression in 40 and 35 lesions, respectively, out of 65 samples (Ericsson et al. 2001). Using different microsatellite markers, loss of heterozigocity (LOH) in chromosome 6 including the HLA region, was demonstrated in DNA obtained from uveal melanomas (Metzelaar-Blok et al. 1999). LOH was present in around 20% of the analyzed samples. Retention of heterozigocity was observed in seven out of twenty samples. These data confirm that LOH in chromosome 6 associated with HLA haplotype loss also happen in uveal melanoma. For details see the chapter "altered HLA-I phenotypes".

In contrast to other tumors, the loss of HLA class I molecules in uveal melanoma is not associated with metastatic spread and worse patient survival, but with a favourable prognosis (De Waard-Siebinga et al. 1996; Ericsson et al. 2001). Metastases from uveal melanoma have a preference for a hematogenic spread to the liver and cause a high mortality rate. Blom and coworkers found that "high" HLA class I antigen expression in primary uveal melanoma lesions detected by staining frozen tissue samples with HLA locus-specific mAbs, was correlated with death from metastases (Blom et al. 1997). One interesting possibility is that NK cells can efficiently kill HLA-I negative uveal melanoma clones in the blood circulation, while the HLA class I positive uveal melanoma cells escape and colonize the liver. This hipotesis has been proposed by two independent groups (Blom et al. 1997; Ericsson et al. 2001). This tumor can be a clear example of the anti tumor activity of T and NK cells. The former select HLA-class I negative clones in the primary solid tumor lesion. The later, select HLA class I positive clones during metastatic dissemination via the blood circulation. A similar finding has been reported in colorectal cancer (CRC) where liver metastasis from MSI-H-CRC are HLA-I positive when circulating to liver by the portal vein (Kloor et al. 2010). Metastasis of uveal melanoma and MSI-H CRC represent two independent examples of NK cells selecting HLA-I positive clones when travelling by the blood circulation.

2.1.5 Non Classical HLA Class I Molecules in Tumors

HLA-G, E and F are HLA class I molecules also coded by the genes within the HLA genetic system. They are known as "Non Classical" to be distinguished from classical HLA-A, B and C molecules. Like their classical counterparts they are also composed by a heavy chain covalently linked to the β2 microglobulin (Geragthy 1993). The degree of polymorphism is low with a reduced number of alleles and their function is still partially obscure (Blaschitz et al. 1997; Braud et al. 1998; Llano et al. 1998). It is well stablished that HLA-G can exist in seven different isoforms known to be expressed as membrane-anchored molecules (HLA-G1,G2,G3 and G4 isoforms) or as secreted soluble ones (HLA G5, G6 and G7 isoforms) that are created by alternative splicing. HLA-G interacts with NK cell inhibitory receptors (Rajagopalan and Long 1999; Ugolini and Vivier 2000; Curiliano et al. 2013) and has an important role in inhibiting NK cells (Loke and King 1991; Kovats et al. 1990; Pazmany et al. 1996; Le Boutellier 1997; Le Boutellier and Blaschitz 1999). HLA-G is expressed in the extravillous trophoblast of the human placenta together with HLA-C where HLA-A and B molecules are missing. This peculiar HLA class I tissue distribution is assumed to play an important role in maintaining an immunologicaly priviledged site where the fetus is protected from the maternal immune response in a semi-allogeneic environment. Some immunologists have proposed that tumor may use similar strategies to escape immune surveillance by loosing HLA-A, B and upregulating HLA-G expression. In this context, it was reported that HLA-G can be aberrantly expressed in human melanoma (Paul et al. 1998). There have been a number of publications demonstrating the analysis of the expression of HLA-G in different tumor tissues, including breast cancer (de Kruijf et al. 2010), hepatocellular carcinoma (Cai et al. 2009), colorectal cancer (Fukushima et al. 1998), renal cell carcinoma (Ibrahim et al. 2001), esophageal squamous cell carcinoma (Ling et al. 2011), lung cancer (Urosevic et al. 2001), and ovarian cancer (Sheu and Shih 2007). A recent review by Zhang and coworkers summarizes these data on HLA-G expression in different ypes of cancer (Zhang et al. 2018).

We did an extensive analysis looking for HLA-G cell surface expression in fifty cryopreserved human tumor tissues of different origin and thirty one tumor cell lines using three different monoclonal antibodies. We found that different HLA-G isoforms were transcribed with different intensity in most of the tumor samples studied, but we did not detect HLA-G at the tumor cell surface (Real et al. 1999a, b). Similar results were reported by other groups. Davies and coworkers did not detect HLA-G protein expression using immunohistological analysis of a large number of frozen tissue sections from different types of tumors and several tumor cell lines by flow cytometry (Davies et al. 2001). Frumento et al. analyzed 45 melanoma cell lines before and after IFNγ treatment by flow cytometry and 8 melanoma tumor tissues by immunohistochemistry and no evidence of HLA-G cell surface expression was found (Frumento et al. 2000). Pangault and coworkers also indicated that HLA-G protein expression is not induced during malignant transformation (Pangault et al. 1999). Polakova et al reported that HLA-G is not expressed in freshly isolated human leukemia cells (Polakova et al. 2003). These data suggest that HLA-G is transcribed and translated in a large variety of tumor cell lines and neoplastic tissues but the cell surface expression is rare possibily due to a strong negative post-transcriptional control (Real et al. 1999a; Davies et al. 2001; Frumento et al. 2000). In our studies, HLA-G was clearly detected in JEG-3 choriocarcinoma cell line and in the histiocytic lymphoma U-937 using flow cytometry technique (Real et al. 1999a). The controversies in the data obtained on HLA-G in tumors by different groups have not yet been solved (Chang and Ferrone 2003). It is possible that these different results might be due to the use of paraffin embedded "versus" cryopreserved tumor tissues and the use of anti HLA-G antibodies that do not distinguish between intracytoplasmic and cell surface expression. It is important to remember that tumor escape variants that loose the expression of the T cell restriction element (one HLA-A,B,C allele) and at the same time express the NK cell inhibitory molecules, such as HLA-G, are going to be selected. However, in most cases HLA-G has been analyzed without evaluation of the expression of HLA A,B,C in the same tumor sample.

HLA-E is another non-classical HLA class I molecule, which aslo became very attractive for tumor immunologist when they had discovered that surface expression of HLA-E depends on the binding of conserved peptides from different HLA-A, B, C molecules, including HLA-G and that HLA-E is involved in the inhibition of NK cell mediated cytolysis by interacting with the lectin-type derived NK inhibitory receptor CD94/NKG2A (Braud et al. 1997, 1998; Lee et al. 1998). We have studied the possible aberrant expression of HLA-E in human tumors in cooperation with Daniel Geragthy (Fred Hutchinson Cancer Research Center, Seattle, USA) (Marin et al. 2003). We found that HLA-E was mainly detected in leukemia derived cell lines and in

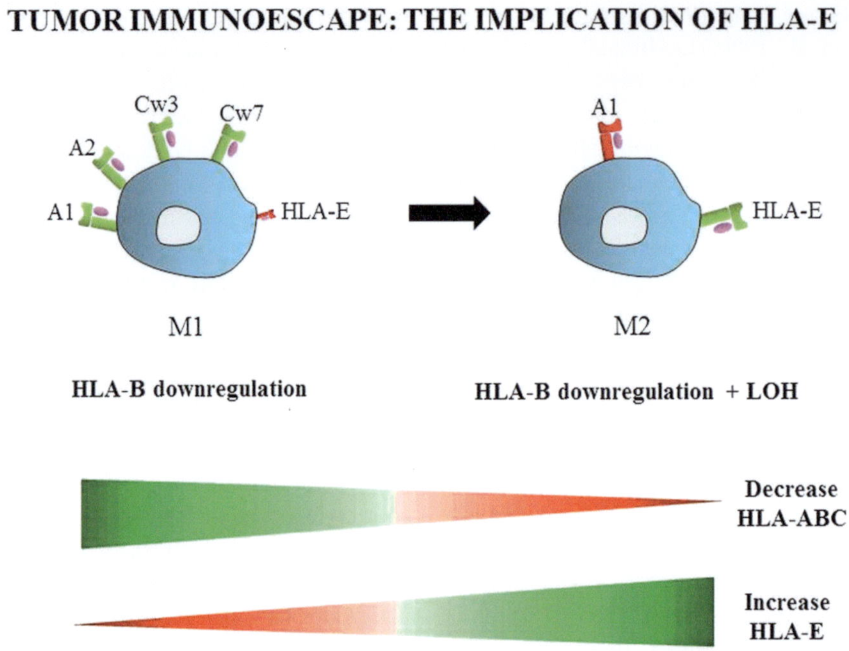

Fig. 2.21 Melanoma cell line M1 was derived from a primary tumor of a melanoma patient. Line M1 shows HLA-B locus loss. Cell line M2 was obtained by immunoselection "in vitro" from M1 using HLA-A2 restricted CTL clone. M2 show a combination of HLA haplotype and HLA-B locus loss. Both cell lines were obtained from Dr Jesper Zeuthen of the Danish Cancer Center (Copenhagen, Denmark). M2 express a single HLA-A allele and HLA-E. Selective loss of HLA-Ia molecules was accompanied by an increased cell surface expression of HLA-E. Similar results were obtained the cervical cell line 808. (See Marin et al. 2003 and Real et al. 1998)

tumour cell lines of different origin showing an imbalance in heavy chain/β2m expression, i.e. a reduced HLA class Ia expression with an increased cell surface level of HLA-E. For instance, a cervical tumor cell line 808 and a melanoma cell line R22.2 expressing a single HLA-A1 allele, also expressed HLA-E (Brady et al. 2000; Marin et al. 2003).There was no HLA-E cell surface expression in tumor cell lines with total loss of HLA class Ia expression, including cell lines with low transcription of HLA class I heavy chains or with β2m mutations. Our findings suggest that HLA-E expression can be detected only in a limited number of tumor cell lines with peculiar phenotypic and genotypic characteristics, such as HLA class Ia downregulation and free β2 microglobulin. The aberrant HLA-E expression might be of particular relevance in HLA tumor phenotypes that express a single HLA-A allele when NK inhibition is markedly reduced due to the downregulation of HLA-B and C alleles (Marin et al. 2003). Figure 2.21 shows an example of two melanoma metastases from the same patient (M1 and M2) which during cancer progression lost all HLA-Ia alleles except HLA-A1 and increased HLA-E expression.

2.2 MHC/HLA Class I Expression in Metastasis

It has been known for many years that metastatic process is a highly complex biological phenomenon that results in colonization of different organs and tissues of the body by tumor cells derived from the primary tumor (Fidler and Kripke 1977). Tumor clones from primary lesions can detach from solid tumor mass, invade the surrounding tissue by destroying the basal membrane and start to migrate to nearby or to distant organs. Metastatic colonization is not random and the classical idea of "seed and soil" is a hypothesis suggesting that there are multiple molecular patterns governing this distant colonization (Zeidman 1957; Kripke et al. 1978). Cellular immune system also plays an important role in controlling metastatic spread via blood circulation or by the lymphatic vessels and lymph nodes. T lymphocytes and NK cells are the leading cellular effectors able to control metastatic spread and both are deeply influenced by the level of MHC-I expression in metastatic cancer cells (Eisenbach et al. 1983; Hammerling et al. 1986; Ljunggren and Karre 1986; Perez et al. 1990; Garrido and Klein 1991a, b; Garcia-Lora et al. 2001).

Metastatic colonies in mice and humans can have the same or different H-2 class I phenotype as the original tumor clone (Ruiz-Cabello et al. 1989; Perez et al. 1990; Garrido and Algarra 2001; Romero et al. 2018). Indeed, it is possible to detect MHC class I positive and negative metastatic colonies in mouse models what makes it difficult to understand the escape route of a particular metastatic tumor cell. Similarly, changes in the HLA-I tumor phenotypes can also be detected in metastases derived from human tumors, but the information available is still very limited and comes predominantely from the investigation of melanoma and colorectal carcinoma (Natali et al. 1983b; Lopez-Nevot et al. 1989, Cordon-Cardo et al. 1991; Mendez et al. 2006; Carretero et al. 2008; Kloor et al. 2010). It is, therefore, not easy to have a clear picture of altered HLA-I profiles used by metastatic tumour cells to escape T and NK cell responses. Furthermore, the routes used by tumor cells to migrate to distant tissues (blood or lymph nodes) are greately influenced by the immune effector mechanisms used by the host to fight this dissemination and is very much related to the HLA-I profiles observed in metastatic tumor cells.

In the first section of this chapter I have summarized the present knowledge on MHC class I expression in "Spontaneous Metastasis" obtained in my laboratory in Granada as a result of the investigation of the methylcholantrene induced fibrosarcoma: the "GR9" tumor system. The second section summarizes the information available on the changes in HLA-I expression during metastatic colonization in humans. Finally, I have also analyzed and discussed the interesting phenomenon of "Metastatic Dormancy" that was clearly demonstrated and reproduced in a particular H-2 class-I negative tumor clone of the "GR9" methylcholantrene induced fibrosarcoma. "Dormancy" is also related to the level of MHC expression.

2.2.1 H-2 Class I Expression in Spontaneous Metastases in Mice

In experimental models it is possible to simulate the phenomenon of metastatic spread observed in the clinical setting in humans. The "spontaneous metastasis assay" is frequently used in inbread mice (see Fig. 2.22) and is induced by a subcutaneous inyection of syngeneic tumor cells into the footpad of a mouse. After a short period of time that depends on different factors, such as the number of inoculated cells or tumor antigenicity, the local primary tumor will start growing and when it reaches 10 mm will be removed. In several weeks the mouse will be analyzed for the presence of distant metastasis in different organs (lung, liver, lymph nodes ...etc.). Metastatic colonies can be isolated and adapted to cell culture for further laboratory analysis. This assay has been widely used and is the one that resembles the natural history of metastatic colonization in cancer patients (Romero et al. 2018). The B16 melanoma which originated spontaneously in a C57/Bl6 mouse in 1954 was obtained from the Jackson Laboratory, Bar harbor, Maine in 1970 and was extensively analyzed by Isaiah Fidler (Fidler 1970, 1973, 1975). B16 melanoma is the most widely used mouse model of metastasis.

We know from our studies with the mouse fibrosarcoma GR9 that different tumor clones present in the primary tumor have different H-2 class I expression and different metastatic capacities ranging from high to low (Perez et al. 1990; Algarra et al. 1991; Garcia-Lora et al. 2001, 2003a; Garrido et al. 2016b). Metastatic

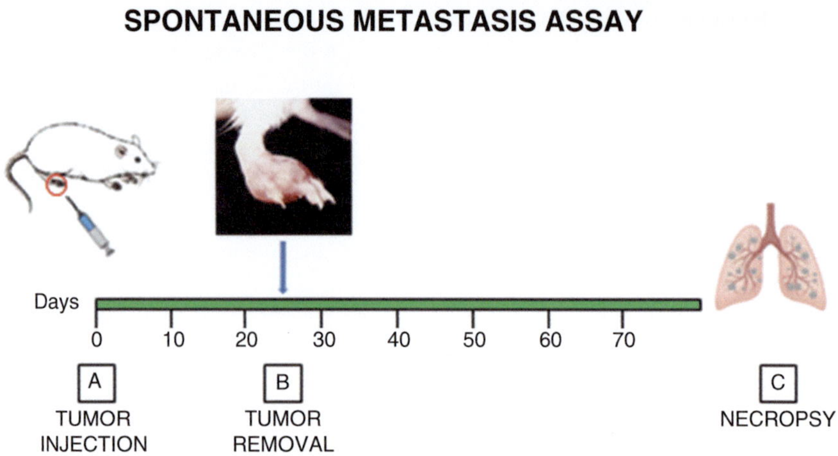

Fig. 2.22 The spontaneous metastasis assay. The assay has three phases: (**a**) the inoculation of the primary tumor cells into the footpad. (**b**) the removal of the primary tumor when it has reached 1 cm in diameter. (**c**) Autopsy of the mouse to detect and isolate metastatic colonies in different organs (lung, liver, lymph nodes…etc)

colonization in our GR9 mouse fibrosarcoma model depends on the amount of H-2 class I molecules expressed by the different clones of the primary tumor. There are clones like A7 that express increased level of H-2 class I molecules and are highly immunogenic with "low" local oncogenicity, however they present "high" metastatic capacity (see Fig. 2.23) (Perez et al. 1990). In contrast, there are other clones, like B9, that are H-2 class I negative with low immunogenicity with "high" local oncogenic potencial and "low" metastatic capacity. All these characteristics are present in the "cocktail of clones" in the primary tumor, where a strong selection mediated by the immune system, by T lymphocytes and NK cells in particular, will take place (Algarra et al. 1989; Garcia-Lora et al. 2001, 2003a).

We also have data indicating that a particular tumor clone present in the primary tumor is capable of generating new mutations in H-2 class I genes during metastatic dissemination producing a "new" level of H-2 heterogeneity. For instance, the mouse primary H-2 class I negative tumor clone B9, can recover all three class I molecules (K, D and L) after IFN treatment. B9 clone is low metastatic and produces only few lung metastasis. We obserbed in these colonies "two" types of H-2 class I metastatic phenotypes: (a) H-2 class I negative with K,D and L genes inducible by IFN treatment, and (b) H-2 class I negative with only K,D genes (but not L) responding to IFN, which suggests that a new mutation (a microdeletion) took place in this metastatic node in the L^d gene. A single primary tumor clone can generate a new H-2 class I diversity during metastatic colonization (Fig. 2.24). We favour the idea that in this tumor model, the L^d molecule presents with the highest affinity the tumor mutated antigen/peptide and therefore there is a strong seletion pressure against this H-2 class I molecule which generates a tumor escape metastatic variant (Garcia-Lora et al. 2001).

Furthermore, we were interested in finding out whether the changes observed in MHC class I expression during tumor development were produced randomly or with a predictable pattern. We injected the GR9-B9 clone (H-2 negative) in different BALB/c mice and analyzed the developed lung metastatic colonies. To our surprise only two H-2 class I phenotypes were observed in different independent experiments: one that could recover K,D and L gene expression after IFN treatment and another type that had L^d gene microdeletion (a "hard" lesion) not inducible by IFN. These findings indicate that H-2 class I alterations observed in metastatic colonies are not random and have particular predictable molecular patterns in a given individual. We

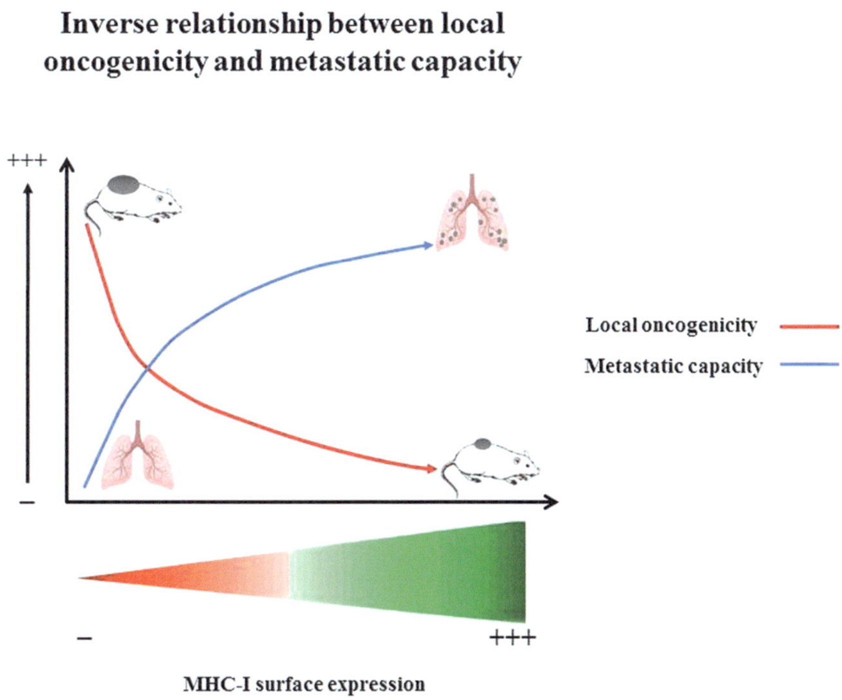

Fig. 2.23 Inverse correlation between H-2 class I expression, local growth and metastatic capacity. H-2 class I positive tumor clones are highly immunogenic and highly metastatic producing a high number of lung metastatic colonies. In contrast, H-2 class I negative mouse tumor clones are low immunogenic and low metastatic and produce only few metastasis in the lung

know that in this mouse metastatic tumor model only these two altered H-2 class I phenotypes derived from a single primary tumor clone will be produced and not other types (Garcia-Lora et al. 2001).

The next question raised was: Is the H-2 expression in metastases originated in immunedeficient mice similar to the one observed in immunocompetent mice? We injected again our B9 clone (H-2 class-I negative) in T cell immuno deficient nude/nude mice. Interestingly, a high number of metastatic colonies were produced and all were now H-2 class I positive (Garcia-Lora et al. 2003a, c). These experiments clearly indicate that T lymphocytes are playing a mayor role in selecting H-2 class I negative metastatic colonies and the absence of the T lymphocyte immune selective pressure allows metastatic cells to growth even though they express H-2 class I molecules.

2.2.2 HLA Class I Expression in Human Metastasis

There are few studies that carefully analyze the HLA-I changes that occurs during metastatic colonization and effors should be made in the future to increase the number of the studied clinical cases. In 1995 Lehmann and coworkers reported a longterm follow up of a melanoma patient. This patient showed different cumulative patterns of HLA-I expression in a series of metastatic lesions in response to T cell mediated immunity. First an HLA haplotype loss, later an additional HLA-B and C locus specific downregulation giving rise to a metastatic cell expressing only one single allele i.e HLA-A24 (Lehmann et al. 1995). These phenotypic changes coincided with different T cell responses directed against different tumor antigens that were presented to T cells by different HLA-I alleles (Ikeda et al. 1997). This study indicates that a cancer cell

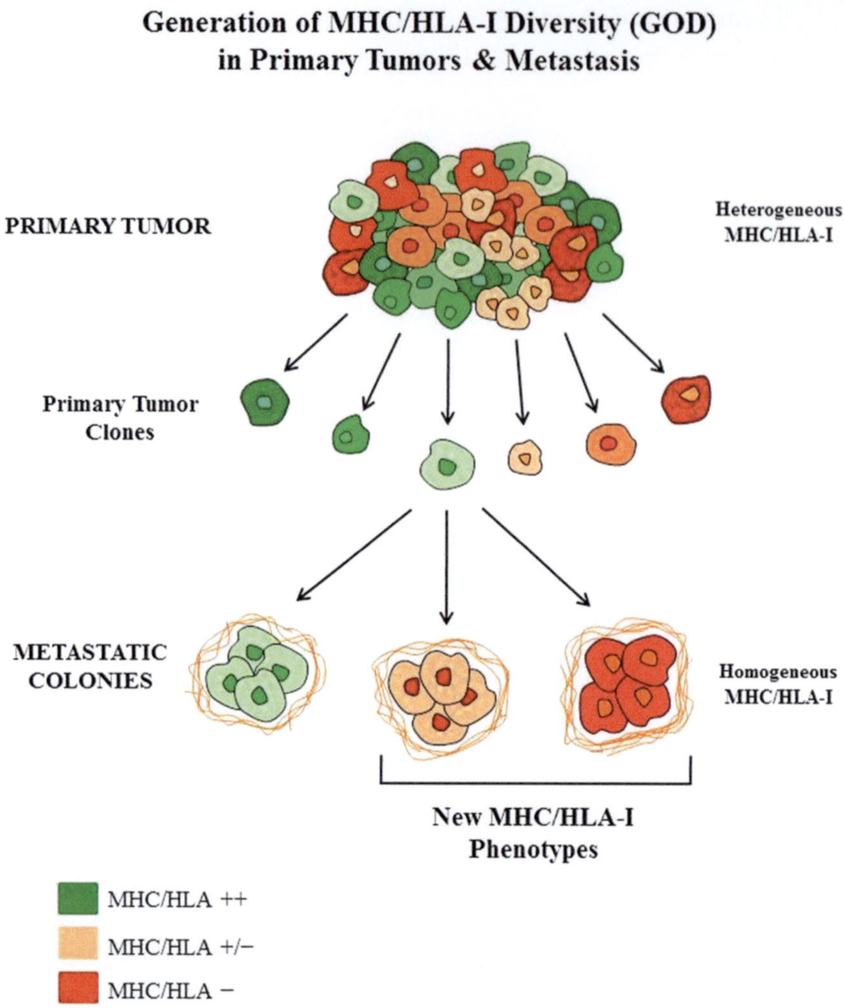

Fig. 2.24 Generation of MHC class I genetic diversity in the primary tumor and metastasis. Primary tumor contains a large variety of clones with different MHC/HLA class I phenotypes: MHC/HLA class I highly positive, intermediate and negative (green MHC/HLA-I positive; red MHC/HLA-I negative). These clones have different metastatic capacity. The metastatic colonies can have the same altered MHC/HLA-I phenotype as the primary tumor or a new one that is not present in the original tumor lesion. In contrast to the primary tumor, the metastatic colonies contain HLA class I homogeneous populations of cells

changes its HLA-I phenotype to escape a particular T cell response and the host changes T cell repertoire to recognize newly emerging tumor escape variants. This dynamic process is impossible to detect in a single metastatic tumor sample obtained from a patient. A decrease in TAP-1 and HLA-I were observed in metastatic versus primary breast cancer (Kaklamanis et al. 1995) and an independent loss of MHC class I and melanocyte differentiation antigen expression was reported in metastatic melanoma favouring the idea in both examples that an "in vivo" immunoselection is taking place (Jager et al. 1997). In 1988–1989 we investigated changes in HLA-I expression in a primary tumors versus autologous metastasis in a variety of tissue samples including laryngeal, colon and gastric carcinomas (Lopez-Nevot et al. 1989). We observed different variants of HLA-I altered phenotypes in primary tumors and metastases: HLA-I positive primary tumor with HLA-I negative metastasis (+/−), HLA-I positive primary tumor/with HLA-I positive metastasis (+/+), negative primary tumor/positive metastasis (−/+), and negative primary tumor with negative metastasis (−/−). These data were obtained using monomorphic anti-HLA monoclonal antibodies and we did not see which alleles were up or down-regulated. However, these observations indicate that a decrease in HLA class I expression during metastatic spread does not always occur. In cooperation with Thierry Boon and Pierre Coulie at the Ludwig Institute in Brussels, we analyzed HLA-I expression melanoma metastasis (cell lines and solid tumor tissue) in two patients that were immunized with MAGE tumor peptides. We showed that these two melanoma lesions were HLA class I negative due to β2 microglobulin mutations and LOH in chromosome 15 (Benitez et al. 1998). These results could explain the failure in the response to the therapeutic vaccination. LOH in chromosome six is a frequent finding in melanoma metastases giving rise to tumour cells expressing only three HLA-I alleles (Mendez et al. 2001).

Similarly to the previously described finding in our fibrosarcoma mouse model, we have observed that multiple metastasis from the same patient can present the same or different HLA-I alterations suggesting that both possibilities are open during the "natural history" of tumor development (Real et al. 2001, Mendez et al. 2001, 2007; Cabrera et al. 2007). In this context, in cooperation with the group of Gustav Gaudernack at the Radium Hospital in Oslo, we have recently observed that a β2 microglobulin point mutation detected in HLA class I negative tumor areas of a primary melanoma lesion appear 16 months later in an homogeneously HLA class I negative lymph node metastasis (see Fig. 2.25). These findings clearly indicate an active ongoing process of T cell mediated immune seletion in this patient (del

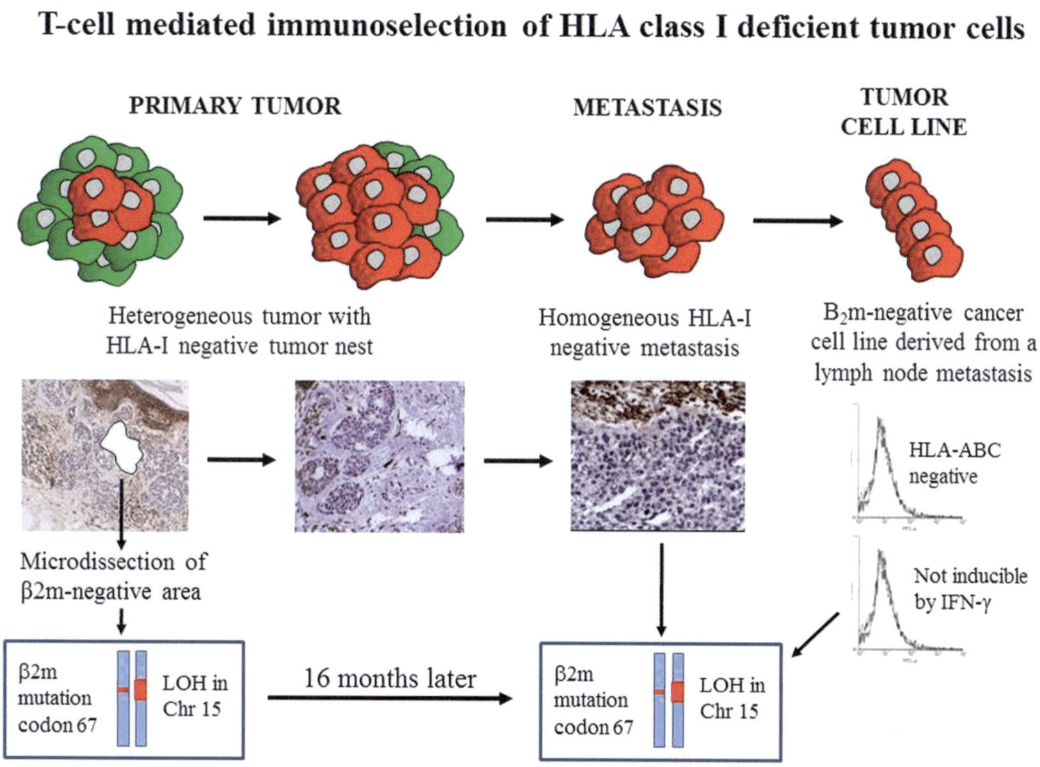

Fig. 2.25 Evidence for T cell immune selection in the metastatic spread in melanoma. The primary tumor is heterogeneous with HLA-I positive and negative areas. A lymph node metastasis obtained 16 months later is homogeneously HLA class I negative with the same point mutation in the β2 microglobulin gene as the primary tumor lesion. (Reprinted by permission of Oxford Publishing Limited, in a Book: Aptsiauri et al. 2014)

Campo et al. 2014). As stated previously, metastatic lesion can be also HLA class I positive (Menon et al. 2004). In this context, Mathias Kloor in Heidelberg have observed that liver metastases from HLA-I negative microsatellite unstable (MSI-H) colorectal cancer are HLA-I positive (Kloor et al. 2010). This interesting observation can be explained by the role that NK cells are playing in eliminating HLA-I negative tumor cells in the portal vein when tumor cells are travelling from the colon tissue to the liver. HLA-I positive tumor cells are NK resistant and can reach the liver tissue and produce metastatic colonies. A similar phenomenon was observed and reported in uveal melanoma metastasis (Blom et al. 1997; Ericsson et al. 2001).

Metastatic ability is influenced by the MHC/HLA phenotype of the tumor cells and also by the immune status of the host. There are different reports indicating that dormant metastases can be awakened after immunosuppressive treatment (Cozar et al. 2008). In this context, we have clearly demonstrated that the MHC class I phenotype of the metastasis can dramatically change if the host is T cell immunodeficient. As previously indicated, the mouse fibrosarcoma tumor clone B9 (H-2 class I negative) produces H-2 class I negative pulmonary metastasis in immunecompetent syngeneic BALB/c mice, which can be recovered by γ-IFN ("soft" lesion). The same tumor clone generates H-2 class I positive metastatic lesion in T cell deficient nude/nude BALB/c mice (Garcia-Lora et al. 2001, 2003a).

I have demonstrated in this chapter that tumor HLA class I loss associated with metastatic colonization is a frequent, but not a common finding (Bandoh et al. 2010; Lopez-Nevot et al. 1989). The MHC/HLA class I phenotype of the metastasis will depend on the route used for spreading i.e. "blood versus lymphatic spread" and also on the molecular lesion responsible for MHC/HLA alteration, i.e. "soft versus hard" lesion. In addition, I have provided examples indicating that new changes in the MHC/HLA class I phenotypes such as new MHC/HLA mutations, that are not present in the original primary tumor clones, emerge during metastatic colonization. Nevertheless, there is very little information about the MHC/HLA class I changes in visceral metastasis in humans due to the difficulty in obtaining such material during the natural history of tumor development.

2.2.3 MHC/HLA Class I Expression and Metastatic Dormancy

There is evidence indicating that tumor cells can remain for long periods of time in the tissues of the host without any clinical syntoms (Aguirre-Ghiso 2007). Some cancer cells neither progress nor are destroyed by the immune system remaining in a "latent" stage of equilibrium with the host tumor microenviroment (Khazaie et al. 1994; Aguirre-Ghiso 2002). This situation of "dormancy" can be changed when the immune status of the host is altered. T lymphocytes are playing a major role in this tumor control (Muller et al. 1998; Romero et al. 2014a). We have reported a clinical case with a pulmonary metastasis of a renal carcinoma immediately after post-transplantation immunosupresive treatment (Cozar et al. 2008) and there are different examples of metastasis appearing many years after the removal of the primary tumor suggesting that the tumor cells and the host can reach a "status quo" of no aggression (Sagalowsky and Molberg 1999).

The MHC class I expression on the tumor cell also play a role in dormancy. We have obtained evidence that our mouse fibrosarcoma tumor clone (GR9-B11) can remain for a long period of time (24 months) in a dormant estate after the injection in syngeneic BALB/c mice in a spontaneous metastasis assay. These dormant cells awaken after T cell immune depletion of the tumor bearing host (Romero et al. 2014a, b). Metastatic colonies appear in these mice after CD8 and CD4 in vivo depletion (see Fig. 2.1). Interestingly, the sarcoma tumor clone (B11) that induce this phenomenon, is H-2 class I negative with capacity to recover the expression after IFN treatment ("soft" lesion). This same tumor clone produced overt metastasis in T cell deficient mice. GR9-B11 tumor clone is H-2 class I negative but the overt metastasis in T cell depleted mice or in T cell immunodeficient mice are H-2 class I positive. This murine model derived from our GR9 fibrosarcoma induced in a BALB/c mouse (H-2[d]) is so far a unique example obtained in an experimental tumor that can reproduce a stage of dormancy (Romero et al. 2014c). We favour the idea that the potencial for metastatic dormancy is already present in the primary tumor lesion, namely the existence of MHC class I negative tumor clones with very low or now metastatic capacity in immune competent host. Our data clearly indicate that the primary tumor can contain MHC-class I low expressor clones that are poorly metastatic but can produce the phenomenon of dormancy (Romero et al. 2014a, b). The experimental model of dormancy that we have in the GR9 fibrosarcoma with the H-2 negative clone GR9-B11, clearly demonstrate that this phenomenon is associated with an H-2 class I negative phenotype and with the capacity to reexpress H-2 class I molecules ("soft" lesion).

References

Abril E, Mendez R, Garcia A, Serrano A, Cabrera T, Garrido, Ruiz-Cabello (1996) Characterization of a gastric tumor cell line defective in MHC class I inducibility by both alpha and gamma interferon. Tissue Antigens 47:391–398

Abril E, Real LM, Serrano A, Jimenez P, Garcia A, Canton J, Trigo I, Garrido F, Ruiz-Cabello F (1998) Unresponsiveness to interferon associated with STAT1 protein deficiency in a gastric adenocarcinoma cell line. Cancer Immunol Immunother 47:113–120

Aguirre-Ghiso JA (2002) Inhibition of FAK signaling activated by urokinase receptor induces dormancy in human carcinoma cells in vivo. Oncogene 21:2513–2524

Aguirre-Ghiso JA (2007) Models, mechanisms and clinical evidence for cancer dormancy. Nat Rev Cancer 7:834–846

Algarra I, Ohlen C, Perez M, Ljunggren HG, Klein G, Garrido F, Karre K (1989) NK sensitive and lung clearance of MHC class-I deficient cells within a heterogeneous fibrosarcoma. Int J Cancer 44:675–680

Algarra I, Gaforio JJ, Garrido A, Mialdea MJ, Perez M, Garrido F (1991) Heterogeneity of MHC-class-I antigens in clones of methylcholanthrene-induced tumors. Implications for local growth and metastasis. Int J Cancer Suppl 6:73–81

Algarra I, Collado A, Garrido F (1997) Altered MHC class I antigens in tumours. Int J Clin Lab Res 27:95–102

Algarra I, Gaforio JJ, Cabrera T, Collado A, Garrido F (1999) The biological consequences of altered MHC class I expression in tumours. J Biol Regul Homeost Agents 13:90–96

Algarra I, Cabrera T, Garrido F (2000) The HLA crossroad in tumor immunology. Hum Immunol 61:65–73

Algarra I, Garcia-Lora A, Cabrera T, Ruiz-Cabello F, Garrido F (2004) The selection of tumor variants with altered expression of classical and non classical MHC class I molecules: implications for tumour immune escape. Cancer Immunol Immunother 53:904–910

Amiot L, Onno L, Lamy T, Dauriac C, Le Prise PY, Fauchet R, Drenou B (1998) Loss of HLA molecules in B lymphomas is associatedwith and aggressive clinical course. Br J Haematol 100:655–663

Angell TE, Lechner MG, Jang JK, LoPresti JS, Epstein AL (2014) MHC class I loss is a frequent mechanism of immune escape in papillary thyroid cancer that is reversed by interferon and selumetinib treatment in vitro. Clin Cancer Res 20:6034–6044

Aptsiauri N et al (2007) MHC class I antigens and immune surveillance in transformed cells. Int Rev Cytol 256:139–189

Aptsiauri N, Cabrera T, Garcia-Lora A, Ruiz-Cabello F, Garrido F (2008) HLA class I expression, tumour escape and cancer progression. Curr Cancer Ther Rev 5:105–110

Aptsiauri et al (2014) 'Hard' and 'soft' loss of MHC class I expression in cancer cells. In: Rees R (ed) Tumor immunology and immunotherapy. Oxford University Press, Oxford, pp 63–78

Aptsiauri N, Ruiz-Cabello F, Garrido F (2018) The transition from HLA-I positive to HLA-I negative primary tumors:the road to escape from T cell responses. Curr Opin Immunol 51:1–10

Aruga A, Aruga E, Tanigawa K, Bishop DK, Sondak VK, Chang AE (1997) Type I versus type 2 cytokine release by V beta T cell subpopulations determines in vivo anti-tumor reactivity IL-10 mediates a suppressive role. J Immunol 159(2):664–673

Bander N, Yao D, Liu H, Chen Y, Steiner M, Zuccaro W, Moy P (1997) MHC class I and II expression in prostate carcinoma and modulation by interferon-alpha and gamma. Prostate 33:233–239

Bandoh N, Ogino T, Katayama A, Takahara M, Katada A, Hayashi A, Harabuchi Y (2010) HLA class I antigens and transporter associated with antigen processing downregulation in metastatic lesions of head and neck squamous cell carcinoma as a marker of poor prognosis. Oncol Rep 23(4):933–939

Bartholomew JS, Glenville S, Sarkar S, Burt DJ, Stanley MA, Ruiz-Cabello F, Chengang J, Garrido F, Stern P (1997) Integration of high-risk human papillomavirus DNA is linked to the downregulation of class I human leucocyte antigens by steroid hormones in cervical tumor cells. Cancer Res 57:937–942

Benitez R, Godelaine D, Lopez-Nevot MA, Brasseur F, Jimenez P, Marchand M, Oliva MR, van Baren N, Cabrera T, Andry G, Landry C, Ruiz-Cabello F, Boon T, Garrido F (1998) Mutations of the beta2-microglobulin gene result in a lack of HLA class I molecules on melanoma cells of two patients immunized with MAGE peptides. Tissue Antigens 52:520–529

Berah M, Hors J, Dausset J (1970) A study of HLA antigens in human organs. Transplantation 9:185

Bernal M, Ruiz-Cabello F, Concha A, Paschen A, Garrido F (2012a) Implication of the β2-microglobuline gene in the generation of tumour escape phenotypes. Cancer Immunol Immunother 61(9):1359–1371

Bernal M, Garcia F, Concha A, Blanco A, Garrido F, Ruiz-Cabello (2012b) Genome-wide differential genetic profiling characterize CRCs with genetic instability and specific routes to HLA class I loss and immunoescape. Cancer Immunol Immunother. June 61(6):803–816

Bernards R, Schrier PI, Houwelling A, Bos JL, van der Eb EJ, Zijlstra M, Melief CJ (1983) Tumorigenicity of cells transformed by adenovirus type 12 by evasion of T-cell immunity. Nature 305:716–779

Bernards R, Desssain SK, Weinberg RA (1986) N-myc amplification causes down-regulation of MHC class I antigen expression in neuroblastoma. Cell 47:667–674

Berthold F, Hero B, Kremens B, Handgretinger R, Henze G, Schilling FH, Schrappe M, Simon T, Spix C (2003) Long-term results and risk profiles of patients in five consecutive trials (1979–1997) with stage 4 neuroblastoma over 1 year of age. Cancer Lett 197:11–17

Bicknell DC, Rowan A, Bodmer WF (1994) β2 microglobuline mutations: a study of stablished colorectal cell lines and fresh tumors. Proc Natl Acad Sci 91:4751–4755

Bicknell DC, Kaklamanis L, Hampson R, Bodmer W, Karran P (1996) Selection for β2 microglobuline mutation in mismatch repair-defective colorectal carcinomas. Curr Biol 6(12):1695–1697

Bijen C, Bantema-Joppe EJ, Jong R, Leffers N, Mourits M, Eggink H, van der Zee A, Hollema H, Bock G, Nijman H (2010) The prognostic role of classsical and nonclassical MHC class I expression in endometrial cancer. Int J Cancer 126:1417–1427

Blades RA, Keating P, McWillian LJ, George NJ, Stern P (1995) Loss of HLA class I expression in prostate cancer: implications for immunotherapy. Urology 46:681–686

Blaschitz A, Lenfant F, Mallet V, Hartmann M, Bensussan A, Geraghty DE, Le Boutellier P, Dohr G (1997) Endothelial cells in chorionic fetal vessels of first trimester placenta express HLA-G. Eur J Immunol 27:3380–3388

Blom DJR, Luyten GPM, Mooy C, Kerkvliet S, Zwinderman AH, Jager MJ (1997) Human leucocyte antigen class I expression: marker of poor prognosis in uveal melanoma. Invest Ophtalmol Vis Sci 38:1865–1872

Boesen M, Svane IM, Engel AM, Rygaard J, Thomsen AR, Werdelin O (2000) CD8+ T cells are crucial for the ability of congenic normal mice to reject highly immunogenic sarcomas induced in nude mice with 3-methylcholantrene. Clin Exp Immunol 121:210–215

Bonal J, Pareja E, Martin J, Romero C, Garrido F (1986) Repression of class I H-2K, H-2D antigens on GR9 methylcholantrene-induced tumour cell clones is related to the level of DNA methylation. J Immunogenet 13:179–186

Boon T, Cerottini JC, Van den Eynde B, van der Bruggen P, Van Pel A (1994) Tumor antigens recognized by T lymphocytes. Annu Rev Immunol 12:337–365

Brady CS, Bartholomew JS, Burt DJ, Duggan-Keen MF, Glenville S, Telford N, Little AM, Davidson JA, Jimenez P, Ruiz-Cabello F, Garrido F, Stern PL (2000) Multiple mechanisms underlie HLA dysregulation in cervical cancer. Tissue Antigens 55:401–411

Braud V, Allan D, Wilson D, McMichael A (1997) TAP and Tapasin dependent HLA-E surface expression correlates with the binding of an MHC class I leader peptide. Curr Biol 8:1–10

Braud VM, Allan DS, O'Callaghan CA, Söderström K, D'Andrea A, Ogg GS, Lazetic S, Young NT, Bell JI, Phillips JH, Lanier LL, McMichael AJ (1998) HLA-E binds to natural killer cell receptors CD94/NKG2A,B and C. Nature 391(6669):795–799

Breslow A (1975) Tumor thickness, level of invasion and node dissection in stage 1 cutaneous melanoma. Ann Surg 182:572–575

Brouwer RE, van der Heiden P, Schreuder GM, Mulder A, Datema G, Anholts JD, Willemze R, Class FH, Falkenburg JH (2002) Loss or down regulation of HLA class I expression at the alleleic level in acute leukemia is infrequent but functionally relevant and can be restored by interferon. Hum Immunol 63(3):200–210

Browning MJ, Krausa P, Rowan A, Bicnell DC, Bodmer JG, Bodmer WF (1993a) Tissue typing the HLA-locus from genomic DNA by sequence specific PCR: comparison of HLA phenotype and surface expression on colorectal tumor cells. Proc Natl Acad Sci USA 90:2842–2845

Browning MJ, Krausa P, Rowan A, Hill AB, Bicknell DC, Bodmer JG, Bodmer WF (1993b) Loss of human leukocyte antigen expression on colorectal tumors cell lines: implications for anti-tumor immunity and immunotherapy. J Immunother 14(3):163–168

Browning M, Petronzelli F, Bicknell D, Krausa P, Rowan A, Tonks S, Murray N, Bodmer J, Bodmer W (1996) Mechanisms of loss of HLA class I expression on colorectal tumor cells. Tissue Antigens 47(5):364–371

Buckowitz A, Knaebel HP, Benner A, Blaker H, Gebert J, Kienle P, von Knebel DM, Kloor M (2005) Microsatellite instability in colorectal cancer is associated with local lymphocyte infiltration and low frequency of distant metastasis. Br J Cancer 92:1746–1753

Burnet M (1957) Cancer: a biological approach. Br Med J 1:779–786

Burnet FM (1970) The concept of immunological surveillance. Prog Exp Tumor Res 13:1–27

Buszello H, Ackermann R (1994) Immunohistochemical studies on the expression of HLA class I antigens in renal cell carcinoma: Comparison of primary and metastatic tumour tissue. Eur Uro. 25:158–163

Cabrera T, Concha A, Ruiz-Cabello F, Garrido F (1991) Loss of HLA heavy chain and β2 microglobuline in HLA negative tumours. Scand J Immunol 34:147–152

Cabrera T, Garrido V, Concha A, Martin J, Esquivias J, Oliva MR, Ruiz-Cabello F, Serrano S, Garrido F (1992) HLA molecules in basal cell carcinoma of the skin. Immunobiology 185:440–452

Cabrera T, Fernandez M, Sierra A, Garrido A, Herruzo A, Escobedo A, Fabra A, Garrido F (1996) High frequency of altered HLA class I phenotypes in invasive breast carcinomas. Hum Immunol 50(2):127–134

Cabrera T, Salinero MA, Fernandez P, Jimenez P, Canton J, Garrido F (1997) HLA class I alterations in laryngeal tumors. In: Charron D (ed) HLA, genetic diversity of HLA. functional and medical implications, vol I, pp 543–545

Cabrera T, Collado A, Fernandez MA, Ferron A, Sancho J, Ruiz-Cabello F, Garrido F (1998) High frequency of altered HLA class I phenotypes in invasive colorectal carcinomas. Tissue Antigens 52(2):114–123

Cabrera T, Salinero J, Fernandez MA, Garrido A, Esquivias J, Garrido F (2000) High frequency of altered HLA class I phenotypes in laryngeal carcinomas. Hum Immunol 61:499–506

Cabrera CM, Jiménez P, Cabrera T, Esparza C, Ruiz-Cabello F, Garrido F (2003a) Total loss of MHC class I in colorectal tumors can be explained by two molecular pathways: beta2-microglobulin inactivation in MSI-positive tumors and LMP7/TAP2 downregulation in MSI-negative tumors. Tissue Antigens 61(3):211–219

Cabrera T, Lopez-Nevot MA, Gaforio JJ, Ruiz-Cabello F, Garrido F (2003b) Analysis of HLA expression in human tumor tissues. Cancer Immunol Immunother 52(1):1–9

Cabrera T, Pedrajas G, Cozar JM, Garrido A, Vicente J, Tallada M, Garrido F (2003c) HLA class I expression in bladder carcinomas. Tissue Antigens 62:324–327

Cabrera T, Maleno I, Lopez-Nevot MA, Redondo M, Fernandez MA, Collado A, Garrido F (2003d) High frequency of HLA-B44 allelic losses in human solid tumors. Hum Immunol 64:941–950

Cabrera T, Lara E, Romero JM, Maleno I, Real LM, Ruiz-Cabello F, Valero P, Camacho FM, Garrido F (2007) HLA class I expression in metastatic melanoma correlates with tumour development during autologous vaccination. Cancer Immunol Immunother 56(5):709–717

Cai MY, Xu YF, Qiu SJ, Ju MJ, Gao Q, Li YW, Zhang BH, Zhou J, Fan J (2009) Human leucocyte antigen-G protein expression is an unfavourable prognostic factor predictor of hepatocellular carcinoma following curative resection. Clin Cancer Res 15:4686–4693

Campoli M, Ferrone S (2008) HLA antigen changes in malignant cells: epigenetic mechanisms and biologic significance. Oncogene 27(45):5869–5885

Campoli M, Chang CC, Ferrone S (2002) HLA class I antigen loss, tumor immune escape and immune selection. Vaccine 20:A40–A45

Carbone DP (1997) The biology of lung cancer. Semin Oncol 24(4):388–401

Carretero R, Romero JM, Ruiz-Cabello F, Maleno I, Rodriguez F, Camacho FM, Real LM, Garrido F, Cabrera T (2008) Analysis of HLA class I expression in progressing and regressing metastatic melanoma lesions after immunotherapy. Immunogenetics 60:439–447

Carretero R, Cabrera T, Sáenz-López P, Maleno I, Aptsiauri N, Cózar JM, Garrido F (2011) Bacillus Calmette-Guerin immunotherapy of bladder cancer induces selection of human leukocyte antigen class I-deficient tumor cells. Int J Cancer 129(4):839–846

Carretero FJ, Del Campo AB, Flores-Martin JF, Mendez R, Garcia-Lopez C, Cozar JM, Adams V, Ward S, Cabrera T, Ruiz-Cabello F, Garrido F, Aptsiauri N (2016) Frequent HLA class I alterations in human prostate cancer: molecular mechanisms and clinical relevance. Cancer Immunol Immunother 65:47–59

Carretero FJ, Del Campo AB, Zinchenko S, Garrido F, Aptsiauri N (2017) Recovery HLA-A2 and beta2-microglobulin expression in tumor cells using viral vectors. J Cancer Sci Therapy 9:622–629

Catlett-Falcone R, Landowski TH, Oshiro MM, Turkson J, Levitzki A, Savino R, Ciliberto G, Moscinski L, Fernandez-Luna JL, Nuñez G, Dalton WS, Jove R (1999) Constitutive activation of Stat3 signaling confers resistance to apoptosis in human U266 myeloma cells. Immunity 10(1):105–115

Challa-Malladi M, Lieu YK, Califano O, Holmes AB, Bhagat G, Murty VV, Dominguez-Sola D, Pasqualucci L, Dalla Favera R (2011) Combine genetic inactivation of β2 microglobuline and CD58 reveals frequent escape from immune recognition in diffuse large B cell lymphoma. Cancer Cell 20:728–740

Chang CC, Ferrone S (2003) HLA G in melanoma: can the current controversies be solved? Semin Cancer Biol 13:361–369

Chen HL, Gabrilovich D, Virmani A, Ratnani I, Girgis KR, Nadaf-Rahrov S, Fernandez-Viña M, Carbone DP (1996a) Structural and functional analysis of β2 microglobuline abnormalities in human lung and breast cancer. Int J Cancer 67(6):756–763

Chen HL, Gabrilovich D, Tampe R, Girgis KR, Nadaf S, Carbone DP (1996b) A functionally defective allele of TAP1 results in loss of MHC class I antigen presentation in a human lung cancer. Nat Genet 13(2):210–213

Cheng NC, Beitsma M, Chan A, Op den Camp I, Westerveld A, Pronk J, Versteeg R (1996) Lack of HLA class I expression in neuroblastoma is associated with high N-myc expression and hypomethylation due to loss of the MEMO-1 locus. Oncogene 13:1737–1744

Cherif I, Allory Y, Commo F, Gattegno B, Callard P, Paul P (2003) Altered pattern of major histocompatibility complex expression in renal cell carcinoma. Am J Pathol 162, n°2 501-508.

Clark WH, From L, Bernardino EA, Mihm MC (1969) The histogenesis and biologic behavior of primary human malignant melanomas of the skin. Cancer Res 29:705–726

Cochran AJ, Wen DR, Stene M, Fairhurst MV, Hoon DS (1988) Immunobiology of human cutaneous melanoma. Prog Clin Biol Res 256:597–618

Concha A, Cabrera T, Ruiz-Cabello F, Garrido F (1991a) Can the HLA phenotype be used as a prognostic factor in breast carcinomas? Int J Cancer Suppl 6:146–154

Concha A, Esteban F, Cabrera T, Ruiz-Cabello F, Garrido F (1991b) Tumor aggressiveness and MHC class I and II antigens in laryngeal and breast cancer. Semin Cancer Biol 2:47–54

Connor ME, Stern PL (1990) Loss of MHC class-I expression in cervical carcinomas. Int J Cancer 46(6):1029–1034

Cordon-Cardo C, Fuks Z, Drobnjak M, Moreno C, Eisenbach L, Feldman M (1991) Expression of HLA-A,B,C antigens on primary and metastatic tumor cell populations of human carcinomas. Cancer Res 51:6372–6380

Corrias MV, Scaruffi P, Occhino M, De Bernardi B, Tonini GP, Pistoia V (1996) Expression of MAGE-1, MAGE-3 and MART-1 genes in neuroblastoma. Int J Cancer 69:403–407

Corrias MV, Ochino M, Croce M, De Ambrosis A, Pistillo MP, Bocca P, Pistoia V, Ferrini S (2001) Lack of HLA class I antigens in human neuroblastoma cells: analysis of its relationship to TAP and tapasin expression. Tissue Antigens 57:110–117

Cozar JM, Apsiauri N, Tallada M, Garrido F, Ruiz-Cabello F (2008) Late pulmonary metastases of renal cell carcinoma immediately after post-transplantation immunosuppressive treatment: a case report. J Med Case Rep 2:111

Cromme FV, Airey J, Heemels MT, Ploegh HL, Keating PJ, Stern PL, Meijer CJ, Walboomers JM (1994) Loss of transporter protein encoded by the TAP-1 gene is highly correlated with loss of HLA expression in cervical carcinomas. J Exp Med 179:335–340

Csiba AS, Whitwell HL, Moore M (1984) Distribution of histocompatibility and leucocyte differentiation antigens in normal human colon and in benign and malignant colonic neoplasia. Br J Cancer 50:699–704

Curiliano G, Criscitiello C, Gelao L, Goldhirsch A (2013) Molecular pathways: human leucocyte antigen G (HLA-G). Clin Cancer Res 19:5564–5571

D'Alessandro G, Zardawi I, Grace J, McCarthy W, Hersey P (1987) Immunohistological examination of MHC class I and II antigen expression on nevi and melanoma: relation to biology of melanoma. Pathology 19(4):339–346

D'Urso CM, Wang CG, Cao Y, Tatake R, Zeff RA, Ferrone S (1991) Lack of HLA class I antigen expression by cultured FO-1 melanoma cells due to a defect in β2 microglobuline expression. J Clin Invest 87:284–292

Daar AS, Fuggle SV, Fabre JV, Ting A, Morris PJ (1984) The detailed distribution of HLA-A,B C antigens in normal human organs. Transplantation 38:287–292

Davies B, Hiby L, Gardner L, Loke YW, King A (2001) HLA-G expression by tumours. Am J Reprod Immunol 45:103–107

De Jong RA, Boerma A, Boezen HM, Mourits MJ, Hollema H, Nijman HW (2012) Loss of HLA class I and mismacht repair protein expression in sporadic endometroid endometrial carcinomas. Int J Cancer 131(8):1828–1836

De Kruijf E, Sajet A, van Nes J, Natanov R, Putter H, Smit V, Liefers G, van den Elsen P, van de Velde C, Kuppen P (2010) HLA-E and HLA-G expression in classical HLA class I-negative tumors is a prognostic value for clinical outcome of early breast cancer patients. J Immunol 185:7452–7459

De Nooij-van Dalen AG, van Buuren-van Seggelen VH, Lohman PH, Giphart M (1998) Chromosome loss with comcomitant duplication and recombination both contribute most to loss of heterozygosity *in vitro*. Genes Chromosome Cancer 21:30–38

De Waard-Siebinga I, Houbiers JGA, Hilders CGJ, de Wolff-Rouendaal D, Jager MJ (1996) Differential expression of HLA-A and B alleles on uveal melanoma as determined by immunohistology. Ocul Immnol Inflamm 4:1–14

del Campo AB, Kyte JA, Carretero J, Zinchencko S, Mendez R, Gonzalez-Aseguinolaza G, Ruiz-Cabello F, Aamdal S, Gaudernack G, Garrido F, Aptsiauri N (2014) Immune escape of cancer cells with β2 microglobuline loss over the course of metastatic melanoma. Int J Cancer 134(1):102–113

Demanet C, Mulder A, Deneys V, Worsham MJ, Maes P, Claas FH, Ferrone S (2004) Down-regulation of HLA-A and HLA-Bw6 but not HLA-Bw4 allospecificities in leukemic cells: an escape mechanism from CTLs and NK attack. Blood 103(8):3122–3130

Dengjel J, Nastke MD, Gouttefangeas C, Gitsioudis G, Schoor O, Altenberend F, Muller M, Krämer B, Missiou A, Sauter M, Hennenlotter J, Wernet D, Stenzl A, Rammensee HG, Klingel K, Stevanovic S (2006) Unexpected abundance of HLA class II presented peptides in primary renal cell carcinomas. Clin Cancer Res 12:4163–4170

Dong H, Strome SE, Salomao DR, Tamura H, Hirano F, Flies DB, Roche PC, Lu J, Zhu G, Tamada K, Lennon VA, Celis E, Chen L (2002) Tumor-associated B7-H1 promotes T-cell apoptosis: a potential mechanisms of immune evasion. Nat Med 8(8):793–800

Dovhey SE, Ghosh NS, Wright KL (2000) Loss of interferon-gamma inducibility of TAP1 and LMP2 in a renal cell carcinoma cell line. Cancer Res 60(20):5789–5796

Drenou B, Tilanus M, Semana G, Alizadeh M, Birebent B, Grosset JM, Dias P, van Wichen D, Arts Y, De Santis D, Fauchet R, Amniot L (2004) Loss of heterozygosity, a frequent but a non-exclusive mechanism responsible for HLA dysregulation in non-Hodgkin's lymphomas. Br J Haematol 127:40–49

Dunn GP, Sheehan KCF, Old LJ, Schreiber RD (2005) IFN unresponsiveness in LNCaP cells due to the lack of JAK1 gene expression. Cancer Res 65(8):3447–3453

Durrant LG, Ballantyne KC, Armitage NC, Robins RA, Marksman R, Hardcastle JD, Baldwin RW (1987) Quantitation of MHC antigen expression on colorectal tumours and its association with tumour progression. Br J Cancer 56:425–432

Eisen A, Weber B (1998) Recent advances in breast cancer biology. Curr Opin Oncol 10:486–491

Eisenbach L, Segal S, Feldman M (1983) MHC imbalance and metastatic spread in Lewis lung carcinoma clones. Int J Cancer 32:113

Ericsson C, Seregard S, Bartolazzi A, Levitskaya E, Ferrone S, Kiessling R, Larsson O (2001) Association of HLA class I and class II antigen expression and mortality in uveal melanoma. Invest Ophthalmol Visual Sci Vol 42, n°10,2153-2156.

Erlich P (1909) The state of the art of cancer reseach. Ned Tijdschr Geneeskd 5:273–290

Ernstoff MS, Duray P, Stenn K, Kirwood J (1985) Antigenic phenotype of pigment cell lesions: a study of melanoma, its precursor lesions and heterogeneity in metastatic melanoma. J Invest Dermatol 84:430–432

Esteban F, Concha A, Huelin C, Perez-Ayala M, Pedrinaci S, Ruiz-Cabello F, Garrido F (1989) Histocompatibility antigens in primary and metastatic squamous cell carcinoma of the larynx. Int J Cancer 43:436–442

Esteban F, Concha A, Delgado M, Perez-Ayala M, Ruiz-Cabello F, Garrido F (1990) Lack of MHC class I antigens and tumour agresiveness of the squamous cell carcinoma of the larynx. Br J Cancer 62:1047–1051

Esteban F, Redondo M, Delgado M, Garrido F, Ruiz-Cabello F (1996) MHC class I antigens and tumour-infiltrating leucocytes in laryngeal cancer: long-term follow-up. Br J Cancer 74:1801–1804

Eyal A, Levin I, Segal S, Levi I, Klein B, Kuperman O (1990) Variation of HLA-ABC surface antigen expression on adenocarcinoma of the colon in correlation with the degree of differentiation. Nat Immun Cell Growth Regul 9:222–227

Facoetti A, Nano N, Zelini P, Morbini P, Benericetti E, Ceroni M, Campoli M, Ferrone S (2005) Human leucocyte antigen and antigen processing machinery component defects in astrocytic tumors. Clin Cancer Res 11(23):8304–8311

Fearon ER, Vogelstein B (1990) A genetic model for colorectal tumorigenesis. Cell 61(5):759–767

Feenstra M, Rozemuller E, Duran K, Stuy I, van del Tweel J, Slootweg P, de Weger R, Tilanus M (1999a) Mutation in the β2m gene is not a frequent event in head and neck squamous cell carcinomas. Hum Immunol 60(8):697–706

Feenstra M, Veltkamp M, Van Kuik J, Wierstma S, Slootweg P, van Den Tweel J, De Weger R, Tilanus M (1999b) HLA class I expression and chromosomal deletions at 6p and 15q in head and neck squamous cell carcinomas. Tissue Antigens 54:235–245

Feenstra M, Verdaasdonk M, van der Zwan AW, de Weger R, Slootweg P, Tilanus M (2000) Microsatellite analysis of microdisected tumor cells and 6p high density analysis in head and neck squamous cell carcinomas with down-regulated human leukocyte antigen class I expression. Lab Invest 80(3):405–414

Fernandez JE, Concha A, Aranega A, Ruiz-Cabello F, Cabrera T, Garrido F (1991) HLA class I and II expression in rhabdomyosarcomas. Immunobiology 182:440–448

Fernandez MA, Ruiz-Cabello F, Oliva MR, Cabrera T, Jimenez P, Lopez Nevot MA, Garrido F (2000) β2-microglobulin gene mutation is not a common mechanism of HLA class I total loss in human tumors. Int J Clin Lab Res 30:87–92

Ferron A, Perez-Ayala M, Concha A, Cabrera T, Redondo M, Oliva MR, Ruiz-Cabello F, Garrido F (1989) MHC class I and II antigens on gastric carcinomas and autologous mucosa. J Immunogenet 16:413–423

Fidler I (1970) Metastasis: Quantitative analysis of distribution and fate of tumor emboli labeled with ^{125}I-5-Iodo-2-deoxyuridine. J Natl Cancer Inst 45(4):773–782

Fidler I (1973) Selection of successive tumor lines for metastasis. Nature New Biol 242:148–149

Fidler I (1975) Biological behavior of malignant melanoma cells correlated to their survival in vivo. Cancer Res 35(1):218–224

Fidler I, Kripke M (1977) Metastasis results from preexisting variant cells whitin a malignant tumor. Science 197:893–895

Fleming K, McMichael A, Morton JA, Woods J, McGee JO (1981) Distribution of HLA class I antigens in normal human tissue and in mammary cancer. J Clin Pathol 34:779

Frumento G, Franchello S, Palmisano GL, Nicotra MR, Giacomini P, Loke YW, Geragthy DE, Maio M, Manzo C, Natali PG, Ferrara GB (2000) Melanomas and melanoma cell lines do not express HLA-G and the expression cannot be induced by gamma IFN treatment. Tissue Antigens 56(1):30–37

Fukushima Y, Oshika Y, Nakamura M, Tokunaga T, Hatanaka H, Abe Y, Yamazaki H, Kijima H, Ueyama Y, Tamaoki N (1998) Increase expression of human histocompatibility leukocyte antigen-G in colorectal cancer cells. Int J Mol Med 2:349–351

Galon J, Costes A, Sanchez Cabo F, Kirilovsky A, Mlenick B, Lagorde-Pages C, Tosolini M, Camus M, Berger A, Wind P, Zinzindohoue F, Brouneval P, Cugnenc PH, Trajanoski Z, Fridman WH, Pages F (2006) Type, density, and location of immune cells within human colorectal tumors predict clinical outcome. Science 313(5795):1960–1964

Garcia-Lora A, Algarra I, Gaforio JJ, Ruiz-Cabello F, Garrido F (2001) Immunoselection by T lymphocytes generates repeated MHC class I deficient metastatic tumor variants. Int J Cancer 91:109–119

Garcia-Lora A, Martinez M, Algarra I, Gaforio JJ, Garrido F (2003a) MHC class I-deficient metastatic tumor variants immunoselected by T lymphocytes originate from the coordinated downregulation of APM components. Int J Cancer 106:521–527

Garcia-Lora A, Algarra I, Collado A, Garrido F (2003b) Tumour immunology, vaccination and escape strategies. Eur J Immunogenet 30:177–183

Garcia-Lora A, Algarra I, Garrido F (2003c) MHC class I antigens, immune surveillance and tumor immune escape. J Cell Physiol 195:346–355

Garrido F (1987) The biological implications of the abnormal expression of MHC antigens on murine and human tumours. In: David CS (ed) H-2 gene complex: genes, molecules, function, Nato ASI series, vol 144. Plenum Press, pp 623–639

Garrido F, Algarra I (2001) MHC antigens and tumor escape from immune surveillance. Adv Cancer Res 83:117–158

Garrido F, Klein E (1991a) MHC antigen expression I. In: Klein E, Garrido (eds) Experimental tumours. Seminars in cancer biology, vol 2-1. Saunders Scientific Publications, pp 1–2

Garrido F, Klein E (1991b) MHC antigen expression II. In: Klein E, Garrido (eds) Experimental tumours. Seminars in cancer biology, vol 1. Saunders Scientific Publications, pp 1–2

Garrido F, Ruiz-Cabello F (1991) MHC expression on human tumors. Its relevance for local tumour growth and metastasis. Semin Cancer Biol 2:3–10

Garrido F, Schirrmacher V, Festenstein H (1977) Studies on H-2 specificities on mouse tumour cells by a new microradioassay. J Immunogenet 4:15–27

Garrido F, Perez M, Torres MD (1979) Absence of four H-2^d antigenic specificites in an H-2^d sarcoma. J Immunogenet 6(2):83–86

Garrido A, Perez M, Delgado C, Garrido ML, Rojano J, Algarra I, Garrido F (1986a) Influence of class I H-2 gene expression on local tumor growth. Description of a model obtained from clones derived from a solid BALB/c tumor. Exp Clin Immunogenet 3(2):98–110

Garrido ML, Perez M, Delgado C, Rojano J, Algarra I, Garrido A, Garrido F (1986b) Immunogenicity of H-2 positive and H-2 negative clones of a mouse tumour, GR9. J Immunogenet 13(2–3):159–167

Garrido F, Cabrera T, Concha A, Glew S, Ruiz-Cabello F, Stern PL (1993) Natural history of HLA expression during tumour development. Immunol Today 14:491–499

Garrido F, Cabrera T, Lopez-Nevot MA, Ruiz-Cabello F (1995) HLA class I antigens in human tumors. Adv Cancer Res 67:155–195

Garrido F, Ruiz-Cabello F, Cabrera T, Perez-Villar JJ, LopezBotet M, Duggan-Keen M, Stern PL (1997a) Implications for immunosurveillance of altered HLA class I phenotypes in human tumours. Immunol Today 18:89–95

Garrido F, Cabrera T, Accolla RS, Bensa JC, Bodmer W, Dohr G, Drouet M, Fauchet R, Ferrara GB, Ferrone S, Giacomini P, Kageshita T, Koopman L, Maio M, Marincola F, Mazzilli C, Morel PA, Murray A, Papasteriades CRH, Salvaneschi L, Stern PL, Ziegler A (1997b) HLA and cancer: 12th international histocompatibility workshop study. HLA, Genetic diversity of HLA. Functional and medical implications. vol. I. In: Charron D, EDK (eds), pp 445–452

Garrido F, Cabrera T, Aptsiauri N (2010a) “Hard” and “Soft” lesions underlying the HLA class I alterations in cancer cells: implications for immunotherapy. Int J Cancer 127(2):249–256

Garrido F, Algarra I, García-Lora AM (2010b) The escape of cancer from T lymphocytes: immunoselection of MHC class I loss variants harboring structural-irreversible “hard” lesions. Cancer Immunol Immunother 59(10):1601–1606

Garrido C, Paco L, Romero I, Berruguilla E, Stefansky J, Collado A, Algarra I, Garrido F, Lora G (2012) MHC class I molecules act as tumour suppressor genes regulating the cell cycle gene expression, invasion and intrinsic tumorigenicity of melanoma cells. Carcinogenesis 33(3):687–693

Garrido F, Aptsiauri N, Doorduijn E, Garcia-Lora A, van Hall T (2016a) The urgent need to recover MHC class I in cancers for effective immunotherapy. Curr Opin Immunol 39:44–51

Garrido F, Romero I, Aptsiauri N, Garcia-Lora AM (2016b) Generation of MHC class I diversity in primary tumors and selection of the malignant phenotype. Int J Cancer 138:271–280

Garrido F, Perea F, Bernal M, Sanchez-Palencia A, Aptsiauri N, Ruiz-Cabello F (2017) The escape of cancer from T cell-mediated immune surveillance: HLA class I loss and tumor tissue architecture. Vaccines 5:7. https://doi.org/10.3390/vaccines5010007

Garrido MA, Rodriguez T, Zinchenko S, Maleno I, Ruiz-Cabello F, Concha A, Olea N, Garrido F, Aptsiauri N (2018) HLA-I alterations in breast carcinoma are associated with a high frequency of the loss of heterozygosity at chromosome 6 and 15. Immunogenetics. https://doi.org/10.1007/s00251-018-1074-2

Geragthy D (1993) Structure of the HLA class I region and expression of its resident genes. Curr Opin Immunol 5:3–7

Giannakis M, Mu XJ, Shukla SA, Qian ZR, Cohen O, Nishihara R, Bahl S, Cao Y, Amin-Mansour A, Yamauchi M, Sukawa Y, Stewart C, Rosenberg M, Mima K et al (2016) Genomic correlates of immune-cell infiltrates in colorectal carcinoma. Cell Rep 15:857–865

Gleason DF, Mellinger GT (1974) Prediction of prognosis for prostatic adenocarcinoma by combined histological grading and clinical staging. J Urol 111(1):58–64

Goeppert B, Frauenschuh L, Zucknick M, Stenzinger A, Andrulis M, Klauschen F, Joehrens K, Warth A, Renner M, Mehrabi A, Hafezi M, Thelen A, Schirrmacher P, Weichert W (2013) Prognostic impact of tumour-infiltrating immune cells on biliary tract cancer. Br J cancer 109(10):2665–2674

Goeppert B, Frauenschuh L, Zucknick M, Roessler S, Mehrabi A, Hafezi M, Stenzinger A, Warth A, Pathil A, Renner M, Schirrmacher P, Weichert W (2015) Major histocompatibility c0mplex class I expression impacts on patient survival and the composition of inflammatory infiltrate in biliary tract cancer. Br J Cancer 113(9):1343–1349

Grandis JR, Falkner DM, Melhem MF, Gooding WE, Drenning SD, Morel PA (2000) Human leukocyte antigen class I allelic and haplotype loss in squamous cell carcinoma of the head and neck: clinical and immunogenetic consequences. Clin Cancer Res 6(7):2794–2802

Grasso C, Giannakis M, Wells D, Hamada T, Mu X et al (2018) Genetic mechanisms of immune evasion in colorectal cancer. Cancer Discovery. https://doi.org/10.1158/2159-8290.CD-17-1327

Gutierrez J, Lopez-Nevot MA, Cabrera T, Oliva R, Esquivias J, Ruiz-Cabello, Garrido F (1987) Class I and II HLA antigen distribution in normal mucosa, adenoma and colon carcinoma: relation with malignancy and invasiveness. Exp Clin Immunogenet 4:144–152

Hammerling G, Klar D, Katzav S, Segal S, Feldman M, Wallich R, Hammerling A (1986) Manipulation of metastasis and tumor growth by transfection with histocompatibility class I genes. J Immunogenet 13:153–157

Han LY, Fletcher DM, Urbauer DL, Mueller P, Landen CN, Kamat AA, Ling YG, Merrit WM, Spannuth WA, Deavers MT, De Geest K, Gershenson DM, Lutgendorf SK, Ferrone S, Sood AK (2008) HLA class I antigen processing machinery component expression and intratumoral T-cell infiltrate as independent prognostic markers in ovarian carcinoma. Clin Cancer Res 14(11):3372–3379

Hicklin DJ, Wang Z, Arienti F, Rivoltini L, Parmiani G, Ferrone S (1998) β2-microglobulin mutations, HLA class I antigen loss, and tumor progression in melanoma. J Clin Invest 101:2720–2729

Hicklin DJ, Marincola F, Ferrone S (1999) HLA class I downregulation in human cancers: T-cell immunotherapy revives an old story. Mol Med Today 5:178–186

Hilders CG, Houbiers JG, Krul EJ, Fleuren GJ (1994) The expression of histocompatibility-related leukocyte antigens in the pathway to cervical carcinoma. Am J Clin Pathol 101(1):5–12

Hinz S, Trauzold A, Boenicke L, Sandberg C, Beckmann S, Bayer E, Walczak H, Kalthoff H, Ungefroren H (2000) Bcl-X-L protects pancreatic adenocarcinoma cells again CD95-and TRAIL- receptor mediated apoptosis. Oncogene 19(48):5477–5486

Holzmann B, Bröker EB, Lehmann JM, Ruiter DJ, Sorg C, Riethmüller G, Johnson JP (1987) Tumour progression in human melanoma:five stages defined by their antigenic phenotypes. Int J Cancer 15 39(4):466–471

Hurks HM, Metzelaar-Blok JA, Mulder A, Claas FH, Jager MJ (2000) High frequency of allele-specific down-regulation of HLA class I expression in uveal melanoma cell lines. Int J Cancer 85:697–702

Ibrahim EC, Guerra N, Lacombe MJ, Angevin E, Chouaib S, Carosella ED, Caignard A, Paul P (2001) Tumor-specific up-regulation of the nonclassical class I HLA-G antigen expression in renal carcinoma. Cancer Res 61:6838–6845

Ikeda H, Lethe B, Lehmann F, van Baren N, Baurain JF, de Smet C, Chambost H, Vitale M, Moretta A, Boon T, Coulie PG (1997) Characterization of an antigen that is recognized on a melanoma showing partial HLA loss by CTL expressing an NK inhibitory receptor. Immunity 6:199–208

Imai D, Yoshizumi T, Okano S, Uchiyama H, Ikegami T, Harimoto N, Itoh S, Soejima Y, Aishima S, Oda Y, Maehara Y (2017) The prognostic impact of programme cell death ligand 1 and human leucocyte antigen class I in pancreatic cancer. Cancer Med 6:1614–1626

Ionov Y, Peinado MA, Malkhosyan S, Shibata D, Perucho M (1993) Ubiquitous somatic mutations in simple repeated sequences reveal a new mechanism for colon carcinogenesis. Nature 363:558–561

Ishigami S, Natsugoe S, Nakajo A, Arigami T, Kitazono M, Okumura H, Matsumoto M, Uchicado Y, Setoyama T, Sasaki K, Aikou T (2008) HLA-Class I expression in gastric cancer. Anticancer Res 97:605–608

Jager E, Ringhoffer M, Karbach J, Arand M, Oesch F, Knuth A (1996) Inverse relation-ship of melanocyte differentiation antigen expression in melanoma tissues and CD8(+) cytotoxic T cell responses: evidence for immunoselection of antigen-loss variants in vivo. Int J Cancer 66(4):470–476

Jager E, Ringhoffer M, Altmannsberger M, Arand M, Karbach J, Jäger D, Oesch F, Knuth A (1997) Immunoselection in vivo: independent loss of MHC class I and melanocyte differentiation antigen expression in metastatic melanoma. Int J Cancer 71:142–147

Jager MJ, Hurks HM, Levitskaya J, Kiessling R (2002) HLA expression in uveal melanoma: there is no rule without some exception. Hum Immunol 63:444–451

Jimenez P, Canton J, Collado A, Cabrera T, Serrano A, Real LM, Garcia A, Ruiz-Cabello F, Garrido F (1999) Chromosome loss is the most frequent mechanism contributing to HLA haplotype loss in human tumors. Int J Cancer 83:91–97

Jimenez P, Canton J, Concha A, Cabrera T, Fernandez M, Real LM, Garcia A, Serrano A, Garrido F, Ruiz-Cabello F (2000) Microsatellite instability analysis in tumors with different mechanisms for total loss of HLA expression. Cancer Immunol Immunother 48:684–690

Jimenez P, Cabrera T, Mendez R, Esparza C, Cozar J, Tallada M, Lopez-Nevot MA, Ruiz-Cabello F, Garrido F (2001) A nucleotide insertion in exon 4 is responsible for the absence of expression of an HLA-A*0301 allele in a prostate carcinoma cell line. Immunogenetics 53:606–610

Jordanova ES, Riemersma SA, Philippo K, Schuuring E, Kluin PM (2003) β2-microglobuline aberrations in diffuse large B cell lymphoma of the testis and the central nervous system. Int J Cancer 103:393–398

Kaklamanis L, Hill A (1992) MHC loss in colorectal tumours: evidence for immunoselection? Cancer Surv 13:155–171

Kaklamanis L, Gatter KC, Hill AB, Mortensen N, Harris AL, Krausa P, McMichael A, Bodmer JG, Bodmer WF (1992) Loss of HLA class-I alleles, heavy chains and beta 2-microglobulin in colorectal cancer. Int J Cancer 51:379–385

Kaklamanis L, Townsend A, Doussis-Anagnostopoulou IA, Mortensen N, Harris AL, Gatter KC (1994) Loss of major histocompatibility complex-encoded transporter associated with antigen presentation (TAP) in colorectal cancer. Am J Pathol 145:505–509

Kaklamanis L, Leek R, Koukourakis M, Gatter KC, Harris AL (1995) Loss of transporter in antigen processing-1 transport protein and major histocompatibility complex class I molecules in metastatic versus primary breast cancer. Cancer Res 55:5191–5194

Karamurzin Y, Rutgers JK (2009) DNA mismacht repair deficiency in endometrial carcinoma. Int J Gynecol Pathol 28(3):239–255

Keating PJ, Cromme FV, Duggan-Keen M, Snijders PJ, Walboomers JM, Hunter RD, Dyer PA, Stern P (1995) Frequency of downregulation of individual HLA-A and B alleles in cervical carcinomas in relation to TAP-1 expression. Br J Cancer 72(2):402–411

Kersemaekers AM, Kenter GG, Hermans J, Fleuren GJ, van de Vijver MJ (1998) Allelic loss and prognosis in carcinoma of the uterine cervix. Int J Cancer 79:411–417

Khazaie K, Prifti S, Beckhove P, Griesbach A, Russell S, Collins M, Schirrmacher V (1994) Persistence of dormant tumor cells in the bone marrow of tumor cell vaccinated mice correlates with long-term immunological protection. Proc Natl Acad Sci USA 91:7430–7434

Khong HT, Restifo NP (2002) Natural selection of tumor variants in the generation of "tumour escape" phenotypes. Nat Immunol 3:999–1005

Kikuchi E, Yamazaki K, Torigoe T, Cho Y, Miyamoto M, Oizumi S, Hommura F, Dosaka-Akita H, Nishimura M (2007) HLA class I antigen expression is associated with a favorable prognosis in early stage non-small cell lung cancer. Cancer Sci 98:1424–1430

Kitamura H, Torigoe T, Honma I, Sato E, Asanuma H, Hirohashi Y, Sato N, Tsukamoto T (2006) Effect of human leukocyte antigen class I expression of tumor cells on outcome of intravesical instilation of Bacillus Calmette-Guerin immunotherapy for bladder cancer. Clin Cancer Res 12(15):4641–4644.52-461

Kitamura H, Honma I, Torigoe T, Asanuma H, Sato N, Tsukamoto T (2007) Down-regulation of HLA class I antigen is an independent prognostic factor for clear cell renal cell carcinoma. J Urol i77:1269–1272

Klein B, Klein T, Nyska A, Shapira J, Figer A, Schwartz A, Rakovsky E, Livni E, Lurie H (1991) Expression of HLA class I and class II in gastric carcinomas in relation to pathologic stage. Tumour Biol 12:68–74

Klein B, Levin I, Klein T (1996) HLA class I antigens in human solid tumors. Isr J Med Sci 33:1238–1243

Kloor M, von Knebel Doeberitz M (2016) The immune biology of microsatellite-unstable cancer. Trends Cancer 2(3):121–133

Kloor M, Becker C, Benner A, Woerner SM, Gebert J, Ferrone S, von Knebel Doeberitz M (2005) Immunoselective preasure and human leucocyte antigen class I machinery defects in microsatellite unstable colorectal cancers. Cancer Res 65:6418–6424

Kloor M, Michel S, Buckowitz B, Ruschoff J, Buttner R, Holinski-Feder E, Dippold W, Wagner R, Tariverdian M, Benner A, Schwitalle Y, Kuchenbuch B et al (2007) β2 microglobuline mutations in microsatellite unstable colorectal cancer. Int J Cancer 121:454–458

Kloor M, Michel S, von Knebel Doeberitz M (2010) Immune evasion of microsatelite unstable colorectal cancers. Int J Cancer 127:1001–1010

Koene GJ, Arts-Hilkes YH, van der Ven KJ, Rozemuller EH, Slootweg PJ, de Weger RA, Tilanus M (2004) High level of chromosome 15 aneuploidy in head and neck squamous cell carcinoma lesions identified by FISH analysis: Limited value of β2 microglobuline LOH analysis. Tissue Antigens 64:452–461

Koopman LA, Mulder A, Corver WE, Anholts JD, Giphart MJ, Class FH, Fleuren GJ (1998) HLA class I phenotype and genotype alterations in cervical carcinomas and derivative cell lines. Tissue Antigens 51:623–636

Koopman LA, Van der Slik AR, Giphart MJ, Fleuren (1999) Human leukocyte antigen class I gene mutations in cervical cancer. J Natl Cancer Inst 91:961–975

Koopman LA, Corver WE, van der Slik AR, Giphart MJ, Fleuren GJ (2000) Multiple genetic alterations cause frequent and heterogeneous human histocompatibility leukocyte antigen class I loss in cervical cancer. J Exp Med 191(6):961–976

Korkolopoulo P, Kaklamanis L, Pezella F, Harris AL, Gatter KC (1996) Loss of antigen-presenting molecules (MHC class I and TAP-1) in lung cancer. Br J Cancer 73:148–153

Kovats S, Main EK, Librach C, Stubblebine M, Fisher SJ, DeMars R (1990) A class I antigen, HLA-G, expressed in human trophoblast. Science 248(4952):220

Kripke M, Gruys E, Fidler I (1978) Metastatic heterogeneity of cells from an ultraviolet light-induced murine fibrosarcoma of recent origin. Cancer Res 38:2962–2967

Kruger T, Schoor O, Lemmel C, Kraemer B, Reichle C, Dengiel J, Weinschenk T, Muller M, Hennenlotter J, Stenzl A, Rammensee HG, Stevanovich S (2005) Lessons to be learned from primary renal cell carcinomas: novel tumor antigens and HLA ligands for immunotherapy. Cancer Immunol Immunother 54:826–836

Kurokohchi K, Carrington M, Mann D, Simonis T, Alexander-Miller M, Feinstone SM, Akatsuka T, Berzofsky J (1996) Expression of HLA class I molecules and the transporter associated with antigen processing in hepatocellular carcinoma. Hepatology 23(5):1181–1188

Lampson LA, Whelan JP, Fisher CA (1985) HLA-A,B,C and β2-microglobuline are expressed weakly by human cells of neuronal origin but can be induced in neuroblastoma cell lines by interferon. Prog Clin Biol Res 175:379–388

Lanier LL (2005) NK cell recognition. Annu Rev Immunol 23:225–274
Le Boutellier P (1997) HLA-G: on the track of immunological functions. Eur J Immunogenet 24:397–408
Le Boutellier P, Blaschitz A (1999) The functionality of HLA-G is emerging. Immunol Rev 167:233–244
Le YS, Kim TE, Kim BK et al (2002) Alterations of HLA class I and class II antigen expression in borderline invasive and metastatic ovarian cancers. Exp Mol Med 34:18–26
Lee N, Llano M, Carretero A, Ishitani F, Navarro M, Lopez-Botet M, Geragthy D (1998) HLA-E is a major ligand for the natural killer inhibitory receptor CD94/NKG2A. Proc Natl Acad Sci USA 95:5199–5204
Lee H-W, Min SK, Y-S JU, Sung J, Lim MS, Yang DH, Lee BH (2011) Prognostic significance of HLA class I expressing in gastric carcinoma defined by monoclonal anti-Pan HLA class I antibody, EMR8-5. J Gastrointest Surg 15:1336–1343
Lehmann F, Marchand M, Hainaut P, Puoillart P, Sastre X, Ikeda H, Boon T, Coulie PG (1995) Diferences in the antigens recognized by cytolytic T cells on two successive metastasis of a melanoma patient are consistent with immune selection. Eur J Immunol 25:340–347
Levin MD, Klein T, Goldstein J, Kuperman O, Kanetti J, Klein (1991) Expression of class I histocompatibility antigens in transitional cell carcinoma of the urinary bladder in relation to survival. Cancer 68:2591–2594
Levin I, Klein B, Segal S, Eyal A, Gopas J, Kanetti J, Saadon M, Kuperman O (1992) Expression of HLA class-I encoded cell surface antigens in transitional carcinoma of the urinary bladder. Tissue Antigens 39:19–22
Levin I, Klein T, Kuperman O, Segal S, Shapira J, Gal R, Hart Y, Klein B (1994) The expression of HLA class I antigen in prostate in relation to tumor differentiation and patient survival. Cancer Detect Prev 18:443–445
Ling A, Zhang X, Zhou WJ, Ruan YY, Xu DP, Wang Q, Yan WH (2011) Human leukocyte antigen-G expression is associated with a poor prognosis in patients with esophageal squamous cell carcinoma. Int J Cancer 129:1382–1390
Ljunggren HG, Karre K (1986) Experimental strategies and interpretations in the analysis of changes in MHC gene expression during tumor progression:opposing influences of T cell and natural killer cell mediated resistance. J Immunogenet 13:141–151
Llano M, Lee N, Navarro F, Garcia P, Albar JP, Geraghty D, Lopez-Botet M (1998) HLA-E bound peptides influence recognition by inhibitory and triggering CD94/NKG2 receptors: preferential response to an HLA-G-derive nonamer. Eur J Immunol 28:2854–2863
Lohr J, Ratliff T, Huppertz A, Ge Y, Dictus C, Ahmadi R, Grau S, Hiraoka N, Eckstein V, Ecker RC, Korff T, von Deimling A, Unterberg A, Beckhove P, Herold-Mende C (2011) Effector T cell infiltration positively impacts survival of glioblastoma patients and is impaired by tumor-derived TGF-beta. Clin Cancer Res 17:4296–4308
Loke YW, King A (1991) Recent development in the human maternal-fetal immune interaction. Curr Opin Immunol 3:762–766
Loke YW, Hiby S, King A (1999) Human leukocyte antigen G and reproduction. J Reprod Immunol 43:235–242
Lopez-Nevot MA, Garcia E, Pareja E, Bonal J, Martin J, Ruiz-Cabello F, Serrano S, Garrido F (1986) Differential expression of HLA class I and II antigens in primary and metastatic melanomas. J Immunogenet 13(2/3):219–227
Lopez-Nevot MA, Romero C, Ruiz-Cabello F, Pedrinaci S, Gutierrez J, Oliva MR, Huelin C, Garrido F (1987) Study of class I HLA genes in human tumours. In: Dupont B (ed) X international histocompatibility worshop, histocompatibility testing, New York, pp 473–474
Lopez-Nevot MA, Garcia E, Romero C, Oliva MR, Serrano S, Garrido F (1988) Phenotypic and genetic analysis of HLA class I and HLA-DR antigen expression on human melanomas. Exp Clin Immunogenet 5:203–212
Lopez-Nevot MA, Esteban F, Ferron A, Gutierrez J, Oliva MR, Romero C, Huelin C, Ruiz-Cabello F, Garrido F (1989) HLA class I gene expression on human primary tumours and autologous metastases: demonstration of selective losses of HLA antigens on colorectal, gastric and laryngeal carcinomas. Br J Cancer 59:221–226
Lopez-Nevot MA, Ramal LM, Cabrera T, Ruiz-Cabello F, Garrido F (2002) HLA and cancer: β2-microglobuline mutations and malignant melanoma. In: Zierhut M, Jager M, Ksander B (eds) Immunology of ocular tumours. Swets and Zeitlinger, pp 91–101
Lou Y, Vitalis TZ, Basha G, Cai B, Choi KB, JeVreis AP, Aliott WM, Atkins D, Seliger B, JeVries WA (2005) Restoration of the expression of transporters associated with antigen processing in lung carcinoma increases tumor-specific immune responses and survival. Cancer Res 65:7926–7933
Lu QL, Abel P, Mitchell S, Foster C, Lalani EN (2000) Decrease HLA-A expression in prostate cancer is associated with normal allele dosage in the majority of cases. J Pathol. 190:169–176
MacGranahan N, Rosenthal R, Hiley C, Rowan A, Watkins T, Wilson G, Birback N, Veeriah S, van Loo P, Herrero J, Swanton C, TRACERx Consortium (2017) Allele-specific HLA loss and immune escape in lung cancer evolution. Cell 171:1–13
Madjd Z, Spendlove I, Pinder S, Ellis I, Durrant L (2005) Total loss of MHC class I is an independent indicator of good prognosis in breast cancer. Int J Cancer 117:248–255
Main EK, Monos DS, Lampson LA (1988) IFN-treated neuroblastoma cell lines remain resistant to T cell-mediated allokilling and susceptible to non-MHC restricted cytotoxicity. J Immunol 141:2943–2950
Maiorana A, Cesinaro AM, Fano A, Collina G (1995) Expression of MHC class I and class II in primary breast carcinomas and synchrnous nodal metastases. Clin Exp Metastasis 13:43–48

Maleno I, Lopez-Nevot MA, Cabrera T, Salinero J, Garrido F (2002) Multiple mechanisms generate HLA class I altered phenotypes in laryngeal carcinomas: high frequency of HLA haplotype loss associated with loss of heterozigocity in chromosome region 6p21. Cancer Immunol Immunother 51:389–396

Maleno I, Cabrera CM, Cabrera T, Paco L, Lopez-Nevot MA, Collado A, Ferron A, Garrido F (2004a) Distribution of HLA class I altered phenotypes in colorectal carcinomas: high frequency of HLA haplotype loss associated with loss of heterozygosity in chromosome region 6p21. Immunogenetics 56:244–253

Maleno I, Lopez-Nevot MA, Seliger B, Garrido F (2004b) Low frequency of HLA haplotype loss associated with loss of heterozygosity in chromosome region 6p21 in clear renal cell carcinomas. Int J Cancer 109:636–638

Maleno I, Romero JM, Cabrera T, Paco L, Aptsiauri N, Cozar JM, Tallada M, Lopez-Nevot MA, Garrido F (2006) LOH at 6p21.3 region and HLA class I altered phenotypes in bladder carcinomas. Immunogenetics 58:503–510

Maleno I, Aptsiauri N, Cabrera T, Gallego A, Paschen A, Lopez-Nevot MA, Garrido F (2011) Frequent loss of heterozygosity in the β2-microglobulin region of chromosome 15 in primary human tumors. Immunogenetics 63:65–71

Marin R, Ruiz-Cabello F, Pedrinaci S, Mendez R, Jimenez P, Geraghty D, Garrido F (2003) Analysis of HLA-E expression in human tumors. Immunogenetics 54:767–775

Marincola FM, Shamamian P, Alexander RB, Gnarra JR, Turetskaya RL, Nedospasov SA, Simonis TB, Taubenberger JK, Yanelli J, Mixon et al (1994) Loss of HLA haplotype and B locus down-regulation in melanoma cell lines. J Immunol 153:1225–1237

Marincola F, White DE, Wise AP, Rosenberg SA (1995) Combination therapy with interferon alpha-2a and interleukin-2 for the treatment of metastatic cancer. J Clin Oncol 13:1110–1112

Marincola FM, Jaffe EM, Hichklin DJ, Ferrone S (2000) Escape of solid human tumors from T cell recognition: molecular mechanisms and functional significance. Adv Immunol 74:181–273

Martayan A, Fraioli R, Giorda E, Setini A, Ciccarelli G, Delfino L, Ferrara GB, Giacomini P (1999) Biosynthesis of HLA-C heavy chains in melanoma cells with multiple defects in the expression of HLA-A,B,C molecules. Br J Cancer 80(5–6):639–649

Massucci MG, Torsteindottir S, Colombani J, Brautbar C, Klein E, Klein G (1987) Downregulation of class I HLA antigens of the Epstein-barr-virus encoded latent membrane protein in Burkitt lymphoma lines. Proc Natl Acad Sci (Was) 84:4567–4571

Matsui M, Machida S, Itani-Yohda T, Akatsuka T (2002) Downregulation of the proteasome subunits, transporter and antigen presentation in hepatocellular carcinoma and their restoration by interferon-γ. J Gastroenterol Hepatol 17:897–907

Mattijssen V, de Mulder PH, Schalkwijk L, Manni B, Van't Hof-Grootenboer, Ruiter DJ (1991) HLA antigen expression in routinely processed head and neck squamous cell carcinoma primary lesions of different sites. Int J Cancer Suppl 6:95–100

Mazurenko N, Attaleb M, Gritsko T, Semjonova L, Pavlova L, Sakharova O, Kisseljov F (1999) High resolution mapping of chromosome 6 deletion in cervical cancer. Oncol Rep 6(4):859–863

Mehta AM, Jordanova ES, Kenter GC, Ferrone S, Fleuren GJ (2008) Association of antigen processing machinery and HLA class I defects with clinicopathological outcome in cervical carcinoma. Cancer Immunol Immunother 57:197–206

Meissner M, Reichert TF, Kunkel M, Gooding W, Whiteside TL, Ferrone S, Seliger B (2005) Defects in the human leucocyte antigen class I processing machinery in head and neck squamous cell carcinomas: association with clinical outcome. Clin Cancer Res 11(7):2552–2560

Mendez R, Serrano A, Jager E, Maleno I, Ruiz-Cabello F, Knuth A, Garrido F (2001) Analysis of HLA class I expression in different metastases from two melanoma patients undergoing peptide immunotherapy. Tissue Antigens 57:508–519

Mendez R, Ruiz-Cabello F, Jimenez P, Paschen A, Knuth A, Jager E, Traversari C, Shadendorf D, Boon T, Garrido F (2006) Impact of HLA class I alterations in patients undergoing T cell-specific immunotherapy. 13th IHWC. Immunobiology of the Human MHC. Proceedings of the 13th international histocompatibility workshop and conference. Vol II, IHWC Press, pp 512–514.

Mendez R, Ruiz-Cabello F, Rodriguez T, Del Campo A, Paschen A, Schadendorf D, Garrido F (2007) Identification of different tumor escape mechanisms in several metastases from a melanoma patient undergoing immunotherapy. Cancer Immunol Immunother 56(1):88–94

Mendez R, Rodriguez T, del Campo A, Monge E, Maleno I, Aptsiauri N, Jimenez P, Pedrinaci S, Pawelec G, Ruiz-Cabello F, Garrido F (2008) Characterization o f HLA class I altered phenotypes in a panel of human melanoma cell lines. Cancer Immunol Immunother 57:719–729

Menon A, Tollenaar R, van de Velde CJ, Putter H, Janssen-Van Rhijn CM, Keijzer R, Fleuren GJ, Kuppen PJ (2004) p53 and HLA class I expression are not down regulated in colorectal cancer liver metastasis. Clin Exp Metastasis 21:79–85

Mertens F, Johansson B, Husglund M, Mitelman F (1997) Chromosomal imbalance maps of malignant solid tumors: a cytogenetic survey of 3185 neoplasms. Cancer Res 57:2765–2780

Metzelaar-Blok J, Jager M, Moghaddam PH, van der Slik A, Gighart M (1999) Frequent loss of heterozygosity on chromosome 6p in uveal melanoma. Hum Immunol 60:962–969

Michael A, Pandha HS (2003) Renal-cell carcinoma: tumour markers, T-cell epitopes and potential for new therapies. Lancet Oncol 4:215–221

Moller P, Herrmann B, Moldenhauer G, Momburg F (1987) Defective expression of MHC class I antigens is frequent in B-cell lymphomas of high-grade malignancy. Int J Cancer 40:32–39

Moller P, Mattfeldt T, Gross C, Schlosshauer P, Koch A, Koretz K, Moldenhauer G, Kaufmann M, Otto HF (1989) Expression of HLA-A, B, C, DR, DP, DQ and HLA-D associated invariant chain (Li) in non-neoplastic mammary epithelium, fibroadenoma, adenoma and carcinoma of the breast. Am J Pathol 135:73–83

Moller P, Koretz K, Schlag P, Momburg F (1991) Frequency of abnormal expression of HLA A,B,C and HLA-DR molecules, invariant chain and LFA-3 (CD58) in colorectal carcinoma and its impact on tumor recurrence. Int J Cancer Suppl 6:155–162

Momburg F, Koch S (1989) Selective loss of β2-microglobuline mRNA in human colon carcinoma. J Exp Med 169:309–314

Momburg F, Degener T, Bacchus E, Moldenhauer G, Hammerling GJ, Moller P (1986a) Loss of HLA-A,B,C and *de novo* expression of HLA-D in colorectal cancer. Int J Cancer 37:179–184

Momburg F, Moller P, Moldenhauer G, Hammerling G (1986b) Loss of HLA-A-B-C in colorectal carcinoma is related to the degree of differentiation. J Immunogenet 13:195–199

Momburg F, Ziegler A, Harpprecht J et al (1989) Selective loss of HLA-A or HLA-B antigen expression in colon carcinoma. J Immunol 142:352–358

Montes P, Kerick M, Bernal M, Hernandez F, Jimenez P, Garrido P, Marquez A, Jurado M, Martin J, Garrido F, Ruiz-Cabello F (2018) Genomic loss of HLA alleles may affect the clinical outcome in low-risk myelodysplastic syndrome patients. Oncotarget 9(97):36929–36944

Moore M, Ghosh AK, Johnston D, Street AJ (1986) Expression of MHC class II products on human colorectal cancer: an immunohistological and flow cytometric study. J Immunogenet 13(2/3):201–209

Moore M, Ghosh AK, Jones DJ (1989) MHC status of primary human colorectal carcinoma: biological significance and implications for host immune recognition. Acta Chir Scan Suppl 549:17–25

Morales A, Eidinger D, Bruce AW (1976) Intracavitary Bacillus Calmette Guerin in the treatment of superficial bladder tumors. J Urol 116:180–183

Motzer RJ, Bander NH, Nanus DM (1996) Renal cell carcinoma. N Engl J Med 335:865–876

Muller M, Gounari F, Prifti S, Hacker HJ, Schirrmacher V, Khazaie K, Eblac Z (1998) Tumor dormancy in bone marrow and lymph nodes: active control of proliferating tumor cells by CD8+ immune T cells. Cancer Res 58:5439–5446

Natali PG, Giacomini P, Bigotti A, Imai K, Nicotra MR, Ferrone S (1983a) Heterogeneity in the expression of HLA and tumor associated antigens by surgically removed and cultured breast carcinoma cells. Cancer Res. 43:660–668

Natali PG, Cavaliere R, Ferrone S (1983b) Antigenic heterogeneity of surgically removed primary and autologous metastatic melanoma lesions. J Immunol 130:1462–1467

Natali PG, Bigotti A, Nicotra MR, Viora M, Manfredi D, Ferrone S (1984) Distribution of human class I (HLA-A,B,C) histocompatibility antigens in normal and malignant tissues of nonlymphoid origin. Cancer Res 44:4679–4687

Natali PG, Nicotra MR, Bigotti A, Venturo I, Marcenaro L, Giacomini P, Russo C (1989) Selective changes in expression of HLA class I polymorphic determinants in human solid tumors. Proc Natl Acad Sci USA 86(17):6719–6723

Nie Y, Yang G, Song Y, Zhao X, So C, Liao J, Wang LD, Yang CS (2001) DNA hypermetilation is a mechanism for loss of expression of the HLA class I genes in human esophageal squamous cell carcinomas. Carcinogenesis 22(10):1615–1623

Nouri A, Smith M, Crosby D, Oliver RT (1990) Selective and non selective loss of immunoregulatory molecules (HLA-A,B,C antigens and LFA-3) in transitional cell carcinoma. Br J Cancer 62:603

Nouri A, Hussain R, Oliver R (1994) The frequency of major histocompatibility complex antigen abnormalities in urological tumors and their corrections by gene transfection or cytokine stimulation. Cancer Gene Therapy 1(2):119–123

Ochsenbein AF, Klenerman P, Karrer U, Ludewig B, Pericin M, Hengartner H, Zinkernagel RM (1999) Immune surveillance against a solid tumor fails because of immunological ignorance. Proc Natl Acad Sci USA 96:2233–2238

Ogino T, Shigyo H, Ishii H, Katayama A, Miyokawa N, Harabuchi Y, Ferrone S (2006) HLA class I antigen down-regulation in primary laryngeal squamous cell carcinoma lesions as a poor prognostic marker. Cancer Res 66(18):9281–9289

Pangault C, Amiot I, Caulet-Maugendre S, Brasseur F, Guilloux V, Drenou B, Faucher R, Onno M (1999) HLA-G protein expression is not induced during malignant transformation. Tissue Antigens 53:335–345

Parham P, Barnstable CJ, Bodmer WF (1979) Use of a monoclonal antibody (W6/32) in structural studies of HLA-A,B,C antigens. J Immunol 123:324–328

Paschen A, Mendez RM, Jimenez P, Sucker A, Ruiz-Cabello F, Song M, Garrido F, Schadendorf D (2003) Complete loss of HLA class I antigen expression on melanoma cells: a result of successive mutational events. Int J Cancer 103:759–767

Paterson AC, Sciot R, Kew MC, Callea F, Dusheiko GM, Desmet VJ (1988) HLA expression in human hepatocellular carcinoma. Br J Cancer 57:369–373

Paul P, Rouas-Freisss N, Khalil-Daher I, Moreau P, Riteau B, Le Gal FA, Avril MF, Dausset J, Guillet JG, Carosella ED (1998) HLA-G expression in melanoma: A way for tumor cells to escape from immunesurveillance. Proc Natl Acad Sci 95:4510–4515

Pazmany L, Mandelboim O, Valez-Gomez M, Davis DM, Reyburn HT, Strominger JL (1996) Protection from natural killer cell-mediated lysis by HLA-G expression on target cells. Science 274:792–795

Pellegrino MA, Ferrone S, Reisfeld RA, Irie RF, Golub SH (1977) Expression of histocompatibility (HLA) antigens on tumor cells and normal cells from patients with melanoma. Cancer 40:36–41

Peltenburg L, Schrier P (1994) Transcriptional suppression of HLA-B expression by c-Myc is mediated through the core promoter elements. Immunogenetics 40:54–61

Pera E, Moreno A, Galindo L (1986) Prognostic factors in laryngeal carcinoma. A multifactorial study of 416 cases. Cancer 58:928–934

Perea F, Bernal M, Sanchez-Palencia A, Carretero J, Torres C, Bayarri C, Gomez-Morales GF, Ruiz-Cabello F (2017) The absence of HLA class I expression in non-small cell lung cancer correlates with the tumor tissue structure and the pattern of T cell infiltration. Int J Cancer 140:888–899

Perea F, Sanchez-Palencia A, Gomez M, Bernal M, Concha A, Mendez Garcia M, Gonzalez-Ramirez R, Kerick M, Martin J, Garrido F, Ruiz-Cabello F, Aptsiauri N (2018) HLA class I loss and PD-L1 expression in lung cancer: impact on T cell-infiltration and immune escape. Oncotarget 9(3):4120–4133

Perez M, Garrido A, Algarra I, Garrido F (1985) Different H-2 phenotypes in clones derived from a new BALB/c solid tumor. Its relevance for local tumor growth. Immunologia 4:60–69

Perez M, Cabrera T, Lopez Nevot MA, Gomez M, Peran F, Ruiz-Cabello F, Garrido F (1986) Heterogeneity of the expression of class I and II HLA antigens in human breast carcinoma. J Immunogenet 13:247–253

Perez M, Garrido A, Algarra I, Caballero A, Delgado C, Collado MD, Fernandez-Cruz E, Garrido F (1989) H-2 antigens and tumour associated transplantation antigens in clones derived from a methylcholantrene-induced BALB/c tumour: their influence on the generation in vitro and in vivo of the specific anti-tumour immune response. Exp Clin Immunogenet 6:204–218

Perez M, Algarra I, Ljunggren HG, Caballero A, Mialdea MJ, Gaforio JJ, Klein G, Karre K, Garrido F (1990) A weakly tumorigenic phenotype with high MHC class-I expression is associated with high metastatic potential after surgical removal of the primary murine fibrosarcoma.Int. J Cancer 46(2):258–261

Perez B, Benitez R, Fernandez MA, Oliva MR, Soto JL, Lopez-Nevot MA, Garrido F (1999) A new β2 microglobulin mutation found in a melanoma tumor cell line. Tissue Antigens 53:569–572

Perez-Ayala M, Ruiz-Cabello F, Esteban F, Concha A, Redondo M, Oliva MR, Cabrera T, Garrido F (1990) Presence of HPV 16 sequences in laryngeal carcinomas. Int J Cancer 46:8–11

Polakova K, Krcova M, Kuba D, Russ G (2003) Analysis of HLA-G expression in malignant hematopoetic cells from leukemia patients. Leuk Res 27:643–648

Porgador A, Brenner E, Vadai M, Feldman M, Eisenbach L (1991) Immunization by gamma-IFN-treated B16-F10.9 melanoma cells protects against metastatic spread of the parental tumor. Int J Cancer 6(Supplement):54–60

Rajagopalan S, Long E (1999) A human histocompatibility leukocyte antigen (HLA)-G-specific receptor expressed on all natural killer cells. J Exp Med 189(7):1093–1099

Ramal LM, Maleno I, Cabrera T, Collado A, Ferron A, Lopez-Nevot MA, Garrido F (2000a) Molecular strategies to define HLA haplotype loss in microdissected tumor cells. Hum Immunol 61:1001–1012

Ramal LM, Feenstra M, Collado A, van der Zwan AW, Lopez-Nevot MA, Tilanus M, Garrido F (2000b) Criteria to define HLA haplotype loss in human solid tumors. Tissue Antigens 55:443–448

Real LM, Jimenez P, Canton J, Kirkin A, Garcia A, Abril E, Zeuthen J, Ruiz-Cabello F, Garrido F (1998) In vivo and in vitro generation of a new altered HLA phenotype in melanoma tumor cell variants expressing a single HLA class I allele. Int J Cancer 75:317–323

Real LM, Cabrera T, Collado A, Jimenez P, Garcia A, Ruiz-Cabello F, Garrido F (1999a) Expression of HLA-G in tumours is not a frequent event. Int J Cancer 81:512–518

Real LM, Cabrera T, Canton J, Oliva R, Ruiz-Cabello F, Garrido F (1999b) Looking for HLA-G expression in human tumors. J Reprod Immunol 43:263–273

Real LM, Jimenez P, Kirkin A, Serrano A, Garcia A, Canton J, Zeuthen J, Garrido F, Ruiz-Cabello F (2001) Multiple mechanisms of immune evasion can coexist in melanoma tumor cell lines derived from the same patient. Cancer Immunol Immunother 49:621–628

Redondo M, Ruiz-Cabello F, Concha A, Cabrera T, Perez-Ayala M, Oliva MR, Garrido F (1991a) Altered HLA class I expression in non-small cell lung cancer is independent of c-myc alteration. Cancer Res 51:2463–2468

Redondo M, Concha A, Oldiviela R, Cueto A, Gonzalez A, Garrido F, Ruiz-Cabello F (1991b) Expression of HLA class I and II antigens in bronchogenic carcinomas: Its relationship to cellular DNA content and clinical-pathological parameters. Cancer Res 51:4948–4954

Redondo M, Concha A, Ruiz-Cabello F, Morell M, Esteban F, Talavera P, Garrido F (1997) Class I major histocompatibility complex antigens and tumor ploidy in breast and bronchogenic carcinomas. Cancer Detect Prev 21:22–28

Rees RC, Buckle A-M, Gelsthorpe K, James V, Polter CW, Rogers K, Jacob G (1988) Loss of polymorphic A and B locus HLA antigens in colon carcinoma. Br J Cancer 57:374–377

Rockett JC, Darnton SJ, Crocker J, Matthews HR, Morris AG (1995) Expression of HLA-ABC, HLA-DR and intercellular adhesion molecule-1 in oesophageal carcinoma. J Clin Pathol 48:539–544

Rodolfo M, Luksch R, Stockert E, Chen YT, Collini P, Ranzani T, Lombardo C, Dalerba P, Rivoltini L,

Arienti F et al (2003) Antigen-specific immunity in neuroblastoma patients: antibody and T cell recognition of NY-ESO-1 tumor antigen. Cancer Res 63:6948–6955

Rodriguez F, Peran F, Garrido F, Ruiz-Cabello F (1994) Upmodulation by estrogen of HLA class I expression in breast tumor cell lines. Immunogenetics 39:161–167

Rodriguez T, Mendez R, Roberts CH, Ruiz-Cabello F, Dodi IA, Lopez Nevot MA, Paco L, Maleno I, Marsh SG, Pawelec G, Garrido F (2005) High frequency of homozygosity of the HLA region in melanoma cell lines reveals a pattern compatible with extensive loss of heterozygosity. Cancer Immunol Immunother 54:141–148

Rodriguez T, Mendez R, Del Campo A, Jimenez P, Aptsiauri N, Garrido F, Ruiz-Cabello F (2007a) Distinct mechanisms of loss of IFN-gamma mediated HLA class I inducibility in two melanoma cell lines. BMC Cancer 7:34

Rodriguez T, Aptsiauri N, Mendez R, Jimenez P, Ruiz-Cabello F, Garrido F (2007b) Different mechanisms can lead to the same altered HLA class I phenotype in tumors. Tissue Antigens 69(Suppl 1):259–263

Romero P, Coulie P (2014) Adaptive T-cell immunity and tumor antigen recognition. In: Rees RC (ed) Tumor immunology and immunotherapy. Oxford University Press, Oxford, pp 1–14

Romero JM, Jimenez P, Cabrera T, Cozar JM, Pedrinaci S, Tallada M, Garrido F, Ruiz-Cabello F (2005) Coordinated downregulation of the antigen presentation machinery and HLA class I/b2-microglobuline complex is responsible for HLA-ABC loss in bladder cancer. Int J Cancer 113:605–610

Romero JM, Aptsiauri N, Vazquez F, Cozar JM, Canton J, Cabrera T, Tallada M, Garrido F, Ruiz-Cabello F (2006) Analysis of the expression of HLA class I, proinflamatory cytokines and chemokines in primary tumours from patients with localized and metastatic renal cell carcinoma. Tissue Antigen 68:303–310

Romero I, Martinez M, Garrido C, Collado A, Algarra I, Garrido I, Garcia-Lora A (2012) The tumour suppressor Fhit positively regulates MHC class I expression on cancer cells. J Pathol 227:367–379

Romero I, Garrido C, Algarra I, Collado A, Garrido F, Garcia-Lora AM (2014a) T lymphocytes restrain spontaneous metastases in permanent dormancy. Cancer Res 74(7):1958–1968

Romero I, Garrido F, Garcia-Lora AM (2014b) A novel preclinical murine model of immune-mediated metastatic dormancy. Oncoimmunology 3:e29258. ECollection 2014. Vol 9

Romero I, Garrido F, Garcia-Lora A (2014c) Metastases in immune-mediated dormancy: a new opportunity for targeting cancer. Cancer Res 74(23):6750–6757

Romero I, Garrido C, Algarra I, Chamorro V, Collado A, Garrido F, Garcia-Lora A (2018) MHC intratumoral heterogeneity may predict cancer progression and response to immunotherapy. Front Immunol, article 112. https://doi.org/10.3389/fimmu.22018.00102

Rosa F, Berissi H, Weissenbach J, Maroteaux L, Fellous M, Revel M (1983) The β2-microglobuline mRNA in human Daudi cells has a mutated initiation codon but is still inducible by interferon. EMBO J 2:239–243

Ruiter DJ, Bahn AK, Harrist TJ, Sober AJ, Mim MC (1982) Major histocompatibility antigens and mononuclear inflammatory infiltrate in benign nevomelanocytic proliferations and malignant melanoma. J Immunol 129:2808–2812

Ruiter DJ, Mattijssen V, Broecker EB, Ferrone S (1991) MHC antiegns in human melanomas. Semin Cancer Biol 2(1):35–45

Ruiz-Cabello F, Garrido F (2002) Tumor evasion of the immune system. In: Parmiani G, Lotze M (eds) Tumor immunology: molecular defined antigens and clinical applications. Taylor and Francis, New York, pp 177–203

Ruiz-Cabello F, Ferron MA, Lopez-Nevot MA, Pedrinaci S, Conejo JM, Esteban F, Garrido F (1987) MHC class I antigen expression on human tumors. Histocompatibility Testing. In: Dupont B (ed) X international histocompatibility workshop, New York, p 473, November 1987

Ruiz-Cabello F, Lopez-Nevot MA, Gutierrez J, Oliva MR, Romero C, Ferron A, Esteban F, Hueling C, Piris MA, Rivas C, Garrido F (1989) Phenotypic expression of histocompatibility antigens in human primary tumours and metastases. Clin Exp Metastasis 7:213–226

Ruiz-Cabello F, Perez-Ayala M, Gomez O, Redondo M, Concha A, Cabrera T, Garrido F (1991a) Molecular analysis of MHC class I alterations in human tumour cell lines. Int J Cancer 6(Supplement):123–130

Ruiz-Cabello F, Klein E, Garrido F (1991b) MHC antigens in human tumours. Immunol Lett 29:181–189

Ryschich E, Cebotari O, Fabian OV, Autschbach F, Kleeff J, Friess H, Bierhaus A, Buchler MW, Schmidt J (2004) Loss of heterozygosity in the HLA class I region in human pancreatic cancer. Tissue Antigens 64:696–702

Ryschich E, Notzel T, Hinz U, Autschbach F, Ferguson J, Simon I, Weitz J, Frohlich B, Klar E, Buchler M, Schmidt J (2005) Control of T cell mediated immune response by HLA class I in human pancreatic carcinoma. Clin Cancer Res 11:498–504

Saenz-Lopez P, Gouttefangeas C, Hennenlotter A, Concha A, Maleno I, Ruiz-Cabello F, Cozar JM, Tallada M, Stenzl A, Rammensee HG, Garrido F, Cabrera T (2010) Higher HLA class I expression in renal cell carcinoma than in autologous normal tissue. Tissue Antigen 75:110–118

Sagalowsky AI, Molberg K (1999) Solitary metastasis of renal cell carcinoma to the contralateral adrenal gland 22 years after nephrectomy. Urology 54:162

Sakaguchi S, Sakaguchi N, Shimizu J, Yamazaki S, Sakihama T, Itoh M, Kuniyasu Y, Nomura T, Toda M, Takahashi T (2001) Immunologic tolerance maintained by CD25+ CD4+ regulatory T cells: their common role in controlling autoimmunity, tumor immunity and transplantation tolerance. Immunol. Rev. 182:18–32

Salgado R, Denker C, Demaria S, Sitaine N, Klauschen F, Pruneri G, Wiener S, Van den Eynden G, Baehner FL, Penault-Llorca F, Perez EA, Thompson EA, Symmans WF, Richarson AL et al (2015) The evaluation of tumour infiltrating lymphocytes (TILs) in breast cancer: recommendations by an international TILs working group 2014. Ann Oncol 26:259–271

Sanda MG, Restifo NP, Walsh JC, Kawakami Y, Nelson WG, Pardoll DM, Simons JW (1995) Molecular characterization of defective antigen processing in human prostate cancer. J Nat Cancer Inst 87:280–285

Sarkar AK, Nuchtern JG (2000) Lysis of MYCN- amplified neuroblastoma cells by MYCN peptide-specific cytotoxic T lymphocytes. Cancer Res 60:1908–1913

Schrier P, Versteeg R, Peltenburg LT, Plomp AC, Van't Veer LJ, Kruse-Wolters KM (1991) Sensitivity of melanoma cells lines to natural killer cells: a role for oncogene-modulated HLA class I expression ? Semin Cancer Biol 2(1):73–83

Schultze JL, Nadler LM (2003) Lack of sufficient B7 expression as a tumor escape mechanism: implications for immunotherapy. In: Ochoa AC (ed) Mechanisms of tumor escape from the immune response. Taylor & Francis, London, pp 66–93

Scupoly MT, Sartoris S, Tosi G, Ennas MG, Nicolis M, Cestari T, Zamboni G, Martignoni G, Lemoine NR, Scarpa A, Accolla RS (1996) Expression of MHC class I and class II antigens in pancreatic adenocarcinomas. Tissue Antigens 48:301–311

Seliger B (2012) Novel insights into the molecular mechanisms of HLA class I abnormalities. Cancer Immunol Immunother 61:249–254

Seliger B, Maeurer MJ, Ferrone S (2000) Antigen-processing machinery breakdown and tumor growth. Immunol Today 21(9):455–464

Seliger B, Ritz U, Abele R, Bock M, Tampe R, Sutter G, Drexler I, Huber C, Ferrone S (2001) Immune escape of melanoma: first evidence of structural alterations in two distinct components of the MHC class I antigen processing pathway. Cancer Res. 61:8647–8650

Seliger B, Cabrera T, Garrido F, Ferrone F (2002) HLA class I antigen abnormalities and immune escape by malignant cells. Semin Cancer Biol 12:3–13

Seliger B, Ruiz-Cabello F, Garrido F (2008) IFN inducibility of major histocompatibility antigens in tumors. Adv Cancer Res 101:249–276

Serrano A, Brady CS, Jimenez P, Duggan-Keen MF, Mendez R, Stern P, Garrido F, Ruiz-Cabello F (2000) A mutation determining the loss of HLA-A2 antigen expression in a cervical carcinoma reveals novel splicing of human MHC class I classical transcripts in both tumoral and normal cells. Immunogenetics 51:1047–1052

Serrano A, Tanzarella S, Lionello I, Mendez R, Traversari C, Ruiz-Cabello F, Garrido F (2001) Reexpression of HLA class I antigens and restoration of antigen-specific CTL response in melanoma cells following 5-aza-20-deoxycytidine treatment. Int J Cancer 94:243–251

Sharpe JC, Abel PD, Gilbertson JA, Brawn P, Foster CS (1994) Modulated expression of human leucocyte antigen class I and class II determinants in hyperplastic and malignant human prostatic epithelium. Br J Urol 74:609–616

Shen Y, Zhag J, Miao F, Zhang J, Jiang Q, Chen H, Shan X, Wie W (2005) Relationship between the downregulation of HLA class I antigen and clinicopathological significance in gastric cancer. World J Gastroenterol 11(23):3628–3631

Sheu J, Shih I (2007) Clinical and biological significance of HLA-G expression in ovarian cancer. Semin Cancer Biol 17(6):436–443

Singal DP, Ye M, Bienzle D (1998) Transfection of TAP1 genes restores HLA class I expression in human small-cell lung carcinoma. Int J Cancer 75(1):112–116

Smith MEF, Bodmer W, Bodmer J (1988) Selective loss of HLA-A,B,C locus products in colorectal adenocarcinoma. Lancet 1:823–824

Smith MEF, Marsch SGE, Bodmer J, Gelsthorpe K, Bodmer W (1989) Loss of HLA-A,B,C allele products and lymphocyte-function-associated antigen 3 in colorectal neoplasia. Proc Natl Acad Sci (Washington) 86:5557–5561

So T, Takenoyama M, Mizukami M, Ichiki Y, Sugaya M, Hanagiri T, Sugio K, Yasumoto K (2005) Haplotype loss of HLA class I antigens as an escape mechanism from immune attack in lung cancer. Cancer Res 65(13):5945–5952

Soling A, Schurr P, Berthold F (1999) Expression and clinical relevance of NY-ESO-1, MAGE-1 and MAGE-3 in neuroblastoma. Anticancer Res 19:2205–2209

Soong TW, Hui KM (1992) Locus-specific transcriptional control of HLA genes. J Immunol 149(6):2008–2020

Stern P (1996) Immunity to human Papilloma virus-associated cervical neoplasia. Adv Cancer Res 69:175–211

Sucker A, Zhao F, Pieper N, Heeke C, Maltaner R, Stadtler N, Real B, Bielefeld N, Howe S, Weide B, Gutzmer R, Utikal J, Loquai C, Gogas H, Klein-Hitpass L, Zeschnigk M, Westendorf A, Trilling M, Horn S, Schilling B, Schadendorf D, Griewank K, Paschen A (2017) Adquired IFNγ resistance impairs anti-tumor immunity and gives rise to T-cell-resistance melanoma lesions. Nat Commun 8:15440. https://doi.org/10.1038/ncomms15440

Sugimoto T, Horii Y, Hino T, Kemshead JT, Kuroda H, Sawada T, Morioka H, Imanishi J, Inoko H (1989) Differential susceptibility of HLA class II antigens induced by gamma-interferon in human neuroblastoma cell lines. Cancer Res 49:1824–1828

Terabe M, Berzofsky JA (2004) Immunoregulatory T cells in tumor immunity. Curr Opin Immunol 16(2):157–162

Thomas L (1959) In: Lawrence HS (ed) Discussion of cellular and humoral aspects of the hypersensitivity states. Hoeber-Harper, New York, pp 529–532

Tomita Y, Matsumoto Y, Nishiyama T, Fujiwara M (1990) Reduction of major histocompatibility complex class I

antigens on invasive carcinoma and high-grade transitional cell carcinoma. J Pathol 162:157–164
Torres LM, Cabrera T, Concha A, Oliva MR, Ruiz-Cabello F, Garrido F (1993) HLA class I expression and HPV-16 sequences in premalignant and malignant lesions of the cervix. Tissue Antigens 41:65–71
Torres MJ, Ruiz-Cabello F, Skoudy A, Berrozpe G, Jimenez P, Serrano A, Real FX, Garrido F (1996) Loss of an HLA haplotype in pancreas cancer tissue and its corresponding tumor derived cell line. Tissue Antigens 47:372–381
Tsioulias G, Triadafilopoulos G, Goldin E, Papavassiliou ED, Rizos S, Bassioukas P, Rigas B (1993) Expression of HLA class I antigens in sporadic adenomas and histological normal mucosa of the colon. Cancer Res 53(10 Suppl):2374–2378
Turbitt ML, Mackie RM (1981) Loss of β2 microglobulin from the cell surface of cutaneous malignant and premalignant lesions. Br J Dermato 104:507–513
Ugolini S, Vivier E (2000) Regulation of T cell function by NK cell receptors for classical MHC class I molecules. Curr Opin Immunol 12:295–300
Urosevic M, Kurrer MO, Kamarashev J, Mueller B, Weder W, Burg G, Stahel RA, Dummer R, Trojan A (2001) Human leukocyte antigen G up-regulation in lung cancer associtcs with high-grade histology, human leukocyte antigen class I loss and interleukin-10 production. Am J Pathol 159:817–824
Vago L, Perna SK, Zanussi M, Mazzi B, Barlassina C, Stanghellini MT, Perreli B, Cosentino C, Torri F, Angius A, Forno B, Casucci B, Bernardi M, Peccatori J, Corti C, Bondanza A, Ferrari M, Rossini S, Roncarolo MG, Bordignon C, Bonini C, Ciceri F, Fleischhauer K (2009) Loss of mismatched HLA in leukemia after stem-cell transplantation. N Engl J Med 361:478–488
Vago L, Toffalori C, Ciceri F, Fleischhauer K (2012) Genomic loss of mismatched human leucocyte antigen and leukemia immune escape from haploidentical graf-versus-leukemia. Semin Oncol 39(6):707–715
Van der Bruggen P, Traversary C, Chomez P, Lurquin C, De Plaen E, Van den Eynde B, Knuth A, Boon T (1991) A gene encoding an antigen recognized by cytolitic T lymphocytes on a human melanoma. Science 254:1643–1647
Van Duinen SG, Mauw BJ, de Graaff-Reitsma CB, Ruiter DJ (1984) Immunoelectron microscopic methods for demonstration of antigens on normal melanocytes and other epidermal cells. Lab Invest 50:733–741
Van't Veer LJ, Beijersbergen RL, Bernards R (1993) N-myc suppresses major histocompatibility complex class I gene expression throught down-regulation of the p50 subunit of NF-kappa B. EMBO J 12:195–200
Verheyden S, Ferrone S, Mulder A, Claas FH, Schots R, De Moerloose B, Benoit Y, Demanet C (2009) Role of the inhibitory KIR ligand HLA-Bw4 and HLA-C expression levels in the recognition of leukemic cells by Natural Killer cells. Cancer Immunol Immunother 58(6):855–865
Versteeg R, Kruse-Wlters M, Plomp A, Van Leeuwen A, Stam N, Ploegh H, Ruiter D, Schrier P (1989) Supression of class I human histocompatibility leukocyte antigen by c-myc is locus specific. J Exp Med 170:621–635
Villalobos I, Takahashi Y, Akatsuka Y, Muramatsu H, Nishio N, Hama A, Yagasaki H, Saji H, Kato M, Ogawa S, Kojima S (2010) Relapse of leukemia with loss of mismatched HLA resulting from uniparental disomy after haploidentical hematopoietic stem cell transplantation. Blood 115:3158–3161
Villunger A, Strasser A (1999) The great escape: is immune evasion required for tumor progression? Nat Med 5:874–875
Vitale M, Rezzani R, Rodella L, Zauli G, Grigolato P, Cadei M, Hicklin DJ, Ferrone F (1998) HLA class I antigen and transporter associated with antigen processing (TAP1 and TAP2) down-regulation in high-grade primary breast carcinoma lesions. Cancer Res 15(4):737–742
Vitale M, Pelusi G, Taroni B, Gobbi G, Micheloni C, Rezzani R, Donato F, Wang X, Ferrone S (2005) HLA class I antigen down-regulation in primary ovary carcinoma lesions: association with disease stage. Clin Cancer Res 11:67–72
Vokes EE, Weichselbaum RR, Lippman SM, Hong WK (1993) Head and neck cancer. N Engl J Med 328:184–194
Volgelstein B, Fearon ER, Hamilton SR, Kern SE, Preisinger AC, Leppert M, Nakamura Y, White R, Smits AM, Bos JL (1988) Genetic alterations during colorectal-tumor development. N Engl J Med 319:525–532
Wadee A, Paterson A, Coplan KA, Reddy G (1994) HLA expression in hepatocellular carcinoma cell lines. Clin Exp Immunol 97:328–333
Walboomers JM, Jacobs MV, Manos MM, Bosch FX, Kummer JA, Shah KV, Snijders PJ, Peto J, Meier CJ, Muñoz N (1999) Human papillomavirus is a necessary cause of invasive cervical cancer wordwide. J Pathol 189:12–19
Wang Z, Cao Y, Albino AP, Zeff RA, Houghton A, Ferrone S (1993) Lack of HLA class I antigen expression by melanoma cells SK-MEL-33 caused by a reading frameshift in β2-microglobuline messenger RNA. J Clin Invest 91(2):684–692
Wang Z, Seliger B, Mike N, Momburg F, Knuth A, Ferrone S (1998) Molecular analysis of the HLA-A2 antigen loss by melanoma cells SK-MEL-29.1.22 and SK-MEL- 29.1.29. Cancer Res 58:2149–2157
Wang Z, Marincola FM, Rivoltini L, Parmiani G, Ferrone S (1999) Selective histocompatibility leukocyte antigen (HLA-A2) loss caused by aberrant pre-mRNA splicing in 624MEL28 melanoma cells J. Exp Med 190:205–215
Watson NF, Ramage JM, Madjd Z, Spendlove I, Ellis IO, Scholefield JH, Durrant LG (2006) Immunosurveillance is active in colorectal cancer as downregulation but not complete loss of MHC class I expression correlates with a poor prognosis. Int J Cancer 118:6–10

Whelan JP, Chatten J, Lampson LA (1985) HLA class I and β2-microglobuline expression in frozen and formaldehyde-fixed paraffin sections of neuroblastoma tumors. Cancer Res 45:5976–5983

Whitwell HL, Hughes HPA, Moore M, Ahmed A (1984) Expression of major histocompatibility antigens and leucocyte infiltration in bening and malignant human breast disease. Br J Cancer 49:161–167

Wilson BS, Indiveri F, Pellegrino MA, Ferrone S (1979) DR (Ia-like) antigens on human melanoma cells. J Exp Med 149:658–668

Winchester RJ, Wange CY, Gibovsky A, Kunkel HG, Lloyd KO, Old LJ (1978) Expression of Ia-like antigens on cultured human malignant melanoma cell lines. Proc Natl Acad Sci USA 75:6235–6241

Wintzer HO, Benzing M, von Kleist S (1990) Lacking prognostic significance of beta 2 microglobuline, MHC class I and II antigen expression in breast carcinomas. Br J Cancer 62:289–295

Witjes JA, Umbas R, Debruine FM, Shalken JA (1995) Expression of markers for transitional cell carcinoma in normal bladder mucosa of patients with bladder cancer. J Urol 154:2185–2189

Wölf M, Jungbluth A, Garrido F, Cabrera T, Meyen-Southard S, Spitz R, Ernestus K, Berthold F (2005) Expression of MHC class I, MHC class II and cancer germ line antigens in neuroblastoma. Cancer Immunol Immunother 54:400–406

Xia M, Zhang QJ, ShenYQ XLH, Chen FQ, Miao FQ, Wie W (2007) Concordant expression of proto-oncogene promyelocytic leukemia and major histocompatibility antigen HLA class I in human hepatocellular carcinoma. Tissue Antigens 70:272–282

Yang Y, Zhang J, Miao F, Wei J, Shen C, Shen Y, Xie W (2008) Loss of heterozygosity at 6p21 underling HLA class I downregulation in Chinese primary esophageal squamous cell carcinomas 72:105–114

Yang I, Tihan T, Han SJ, Wrensch MR, Wienke J, Sughrue ME, Parsa AT (2010) CD8+ T cell infiltrate in newly diagnose glioblastoma is associated with long-term survival. J Clin Neurosc 17:1381–1385

Yeung J, Hamilton R, Ohnishi K, Ikeura M, Potter D, Nikiforova M, Ferrone S, Jakacki R, Pollack I, Okada H (2013) LOH in the HLA class I region at 6p21 is associated with shorter survival in newly diagnosed adult glioblastoma. Clin Cancer Res 19(7):1816–1826

Yoshihama S, Roszik J, Downs I, Meissner T, Vijayan S, Chapuy B, Sidiq T, Shipp M, Lizee G, Kobayashi K (2016) NLRC5/MHC class I transactivator is a target for immune evasión in cancer. PNAS 113:5999–6004

Zeidman I (1957) Metastasis: a review of recent advances. Cancer Res 17:157–162

Zhang H, Melamed J, Wei P, Cox K, Frankel W, Bahnson RR, Robinson N, Pyka R, Liu Y, Zheng P (2003) Concordant down-regulation of protooncogene PML and major histocompatibility antigen HLA class I expression in high-grade prostate cancer. Cancer Immunol 3:2–11

Zhang Y, Yu S, Han Y, Wang Y, Sun Y (2018) Human leukocyte antigen-G expression and polymorphisms promote cancer development and guide cancer diagnosis/treatment. Oncol Lett 15:699–709

Zia A, Schildberg FW, Funke I (2001) MHC negative phenotype of disseminated tumor cells in bone marrow is associated with poor survival in R0Mo breast cancer patients. Int J Cancer 93:566–570

HLA Class-I Expression and Cancer Immunotherapy

3

Abstract

The impact of HLA class I loss in cancer immunotherapy is carefully analyzed. Why some metastatic lesions regress and other progress after immunotherapy? Are T lymphocytes responsible for tumour rejection and how these responses can be boosted? These questions are discussed in the context of the molecular mechanisms responsible for MHC/HLA class I alterations. If the metastatic tumour cells harbor "irreversible/hard" HLA lesions, they will escape and kill the host. In contrast, if the molecular lesion is "reversible/soft", tumor cells can potentially recover HLA-class I expression and can finally be destroyed. These important new concepts are integrated together and gain a great importance in the new era of "immune checkpoint antibodies". Finally, the ability to recover HLA-I expression in tumours harboring "structural-irreversible-hard" genetic lesions is seen as a challenge for the future investigation.

Keywords

Cancer immunotherapy · Checkpoint antibodies · HLA class I loss · Recovery HLA-I · HLA gene therapy · HLA-I upregulation · HLA hard alterations · HLA soft alterations · HLA-I mutations · Loss of heterozygosity · Immune selection

Historically cancer immunotherapy has used a variety of biological products that boost T cell responses against tumour cells. For instance, BCG to treat superficial bladder cancer (Morales et al. 1976), Polysacharide K (PSK) for the treatment of gastrointestinal cancer in Asia (Tsukagoshi et al. 1984; Nio et al. 1991), IL-2 and IFN-α (Rosenberg et al. 1987), tumor peptides alone (Marchand et al. 1995, 1999) or loaded in dendritic cells (Nestle et al. 1998) or autologous transfer of T lymphocytes (Andersen et al. 2016) to treat metastatic melanoma. Recently the use of antibodies that regulate T cell cytotoxicity have been approved by the FDA in a variety of metastatic human tumors with encouraging clinical responses (Sharma and Allison 2015; Leach et al. 1996). I favour the idea that a common biological effect of such therapies is the "unblock" of T cell activity followed by the release of TH1 type cytokines in the tumor microenviroment. These cytokines can upregulate MHC/HLA class I expression at the tumor cell surface, restoring the antigen presentation capacity and the restimulation of primed tumor infiltrating T cells. These T cells will encounter again the specific tumour antigen and will induce tumour rejection. These T cells had previously been sensitized by the tumor specific antigen during the natural anti tumor immune response and are now residing in the tumor estroma. Unfortunately, the reason and the mechanism explaining why during cancer immunotherapy some tumor lesions progress while other

F. Garrido, *MHC Class-I Loss and Cancer Immune Escape*, Advances in Experimental Medicine and Biology 1151, https://doi.org/10.1007/978-3-030-17864-2_3

nodes regress is far from being understood (Carretero et al. 2012).

The absence of HLA class I molecules in the tumor cell surface is whithout a doubt a major obstacle for a successfull T cell mediated immunotherapy (Ruiz-Cabello and Garrido 1998; Ruiz-Cabello et al. 2002; Mendez et al. 2006, Thor Straten and Garrido 2016). We have proposed that the progression or regression of a tumor lesion in cancer patients undergoing immunotherapy could be predetermined by the molecular mechanism responsible for the MHC Class I alteration and not by the type of immunotherapy used, i.e.,IL-2, BCG, α-IFN, PSK, tumour peptides, etc… (Garrido et al. 2010a, b). If the molecular alteration responsible for the changes in MHC Class I expression is reversible by cytokines ("soft" lesion), the MHC Class I expression can be upregulated, leading to the activation of the specific T cell-mediated response and tumor regression. However, in case of a structural ("hard" lesion) alteration causing the loss of tumor MHC Class I expression, the escape mechanism will prevail and the primary tumor or metastatic lesion most likely will grow (Fig. 3.1). According to this idea, the nature of the preexisting MHC Class I lesion in cancer cells has a crucial impact determining the final outcome of cancer immunotherapy. See Table 3.1 that summarizes different "soft" and "hard" molecular lesions described in human tumors. See Garrido et al. (2010a) for details.

3.1 Reversible "Soft" Versus Irreversible "Hard" Molecular HLA-I Lesions: Implications for Cancer Immunotherapy

Defects at any step required for the synthesis and assembly of an HLA-I complex can lead to the absence of a particular HLA molecule. Figure 1.3 in page 15 depicts a schematic representation of the antigen processing and presentation pathway, including the HLA synthesis. We have obtained data indicating that the large variety of known mechanisms that can produce HLA-I altered phe-

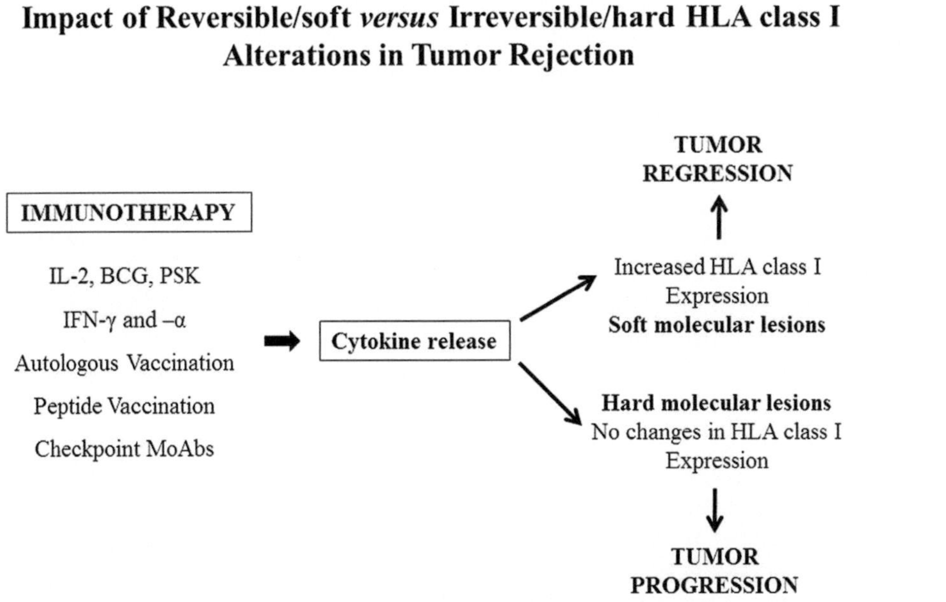

Fig. 3.1 Impact of "hard" and "soft" molecular lesions on cancer immunotherapy. Different types of Immunotherapy can modify the tumor microenviroment and induce the local release of TH type 1 cytokines which can upregulate HLA class I molecules in tumor cells with "reversible/soft" molecular lesions and recover antigen presentation to T lymphocytes and tumour rejection. However, if the molecular lesion is "irreversible/hard" the recovery of HLA class I molecules is unlikely and the metastatic lesion will progress

Table 3.1 Molecular defects underlying MHC Class-I altered expression

Irreversible structural defects	
Chromosome 6	Loss of heterozygosity (LOH)
	HLA haplotype loss
	Mutations of MHC class I heavy chain genes
	HLA allelic loss
Chromosome 15	**Loss of heterozygosity (LOH)**
	β2m gene
	Mutations/deletions
	β2m gene
IFN transduction pathway	Jak-STAT pathway blockade
Reversible regulatory defects	
Transcriptional down-regulation	Coordinated downregulation of HLA A genes
	Coordinated downregulation of HLA B genes
	Coordinated downregulation of HLA C genes
	Coordinated downregulation of heavy chain, β2m and APM molecules
	Coordinated downregulation of antigen- presenting machinery (APM) components
Hypermethylation	MHC class I genes
	Downregulation of HLA-B genes
	Downregulation of HLA class I and APM genes
	Inhibition of the post-transcriptional processing of MHC class I mRNA

notypes can be divided in two groups based on the nature of the alteration and on the possibility to recover tumor HLA expression after the treatment with cytokines (Aptsiauri et al. 2008, 2014; Garrido et al. 2010a, b). Table 3.1 summarizes several "hard" and "soft" molecular mechanisms already defined in human tumors. Mutations or loss of heterozigosity (LOH) associated with macro or micro-deletions in chromosome 6 or 15 are responsible for "hard" lesions. LOH at chromosomes 6 and 15 is frequently found in a variety of human tumors (Maleno et al. 2006, 2011; Garrido et al. 2016). β2 microglobulin mutations are frequently found in melanoma and MSH-I colorectal carcinoma (Bernal et al. 2012; Kloor et al. 2010). In addition, structural "hard" alterations in α or γ-IFN signal transduction pathways have been recently described in association with the lack of MHC/HLA class I upregulation in response to TH type 1 cytoquines released in the tumor microenviroment (Sucker et al. 2017). Different tumor cell lines harbouring such IFN molecular lesions have been reported, althoug the percentage of this type of molecular aberration in solid tumor tissues has yet to be defined. (Rodriguez et al. 2007; Seliger et al. 2008; Abril et al. 1998; Sucker et al. 2017).The recovery of antigen presentation capacity of tumor cells is crucial for restoring anti-tumor T cell mediated cytotoxicity and tumor rejection. Therapies that lead to MHC class I upregulation in MHC-I deficient tumor cells will improve T cell recognition of tumor antigens and clinical responses in immune therapy-based treatment (see Fig. 3.1).

There are several reports indicating that different types of immunotherapy can induce rejection of metastatic colonies with MHC/HLA-I "soft" lesions by locally releasing cytokines such as IFN and upregulating class I expression allowing antigen presentation. For instance, a highly metastatic mouse tumor clone expressing high levels of H-2 class I antigens (GR9-A7) was producing a high number of lung metastatic colonies. Different protocols of immunotherapy administered to the GR9-A7 tumor bearing mice during the spontaneous metastasis assay showed the complete eradication of the lung metastasis (Garrido et al. 2011). Porgador et al showed that immunization with ϒ-IFN treated B16-F10.9 melanoma cells protects against metastatic spread of the parental tumour (Porgador et al. 1991). In this context, we have proposed that T cell based immunotherapy select MHC/HLA-I negative tumor cells with "hard" lesions that cannot upregulate MHC class I molecules and destroy tumor cells with "soft" ones (del Campo et al. 2014a; Garrido et al. 2016). A recent report have shown that an antibody against the Epidermal Growth Factor Receptor (EGFR) induce upregulation of of HLA class I expression on tumour cells (Garrido et al. 2017).

We have obtained data from the study of the patients with superficial bladder cancer treated with BCG showing that post-treatment recurrent tumors have additional "hard" HLA-I alterations associated with LOH at chromosomes 6 and 15 where the HLA region and β2 microglobulin genes are located. Based on these observations we proposed that T cells are responsible for the immune selection and escape of cancer cells with newly acquired additional HLA class I losses. Activation of the immune surveillance after BCG therapy leads to immune selection and elimination of tumor cells with upregulated HLA class I expression and to the outgrowth of cancer cells with HLA class I loss caused by structural alterations (see Fig. 3.2). This hypothesis could explain the higher frequency of LOH in primary tumors of patients with recurrent bladder cancer after BCG treatment, suggesting that tumour cells with "reversible/soft" HLA-I alterations have been eliminated (Carretero et al. 2011; Maleno et al. 2006, 2011).

An interesting observation on a transmissible tumor has been decribed in the Tasmanian devil (Woods et al. 2015). This rare contagious cancer called "Devil Facial tumour Disease" (DFTD) is produced when these animals fight for food. This transmissible cancer has 100% lethality and spreads between these mamals as a facial tumour and has put in danger this species in its natural environment in Australia. A "reversible" immune escape mechanism associated with an epigenetic MHC-I downregulation is responsible for such alterations (Siddle et al. 2013). The absence of MHC class I in the tumor cell surface make it possible the transmission of tumour cells between different "Devils" without an allogeneic immune

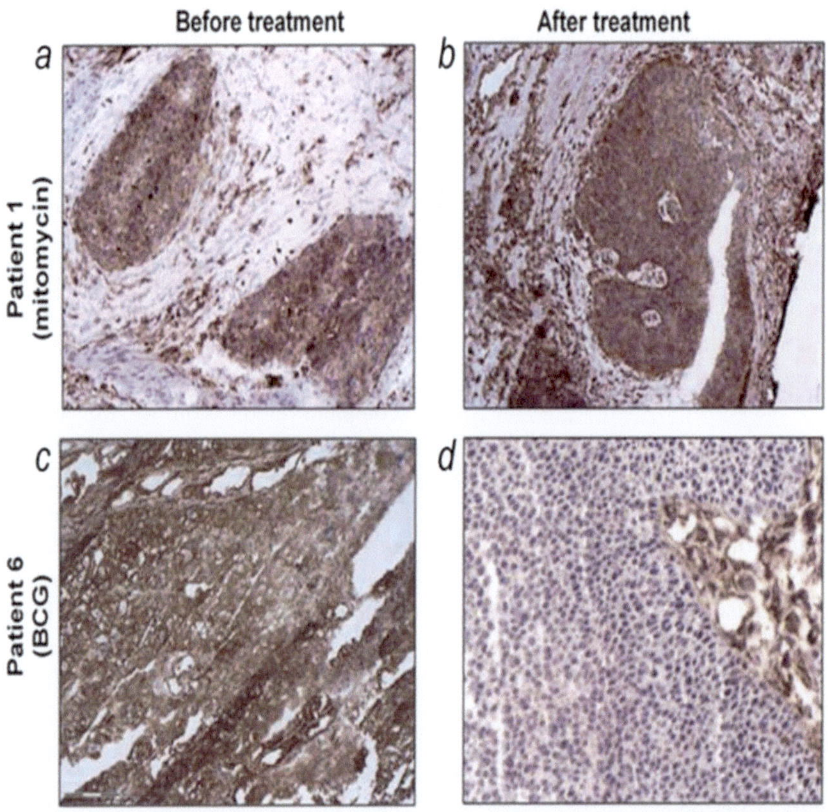

Fig. 3.2 HLA class I expression in bladder cancer tissues before and after mitomicin or BCG treatment. Patient 1 shows positive tumor staining both before (**a**) and after (**b**) mitomycin treatment. In Patient 6, we observed a positive tumor immunolabeling before BCG therapy (**c**) and loss of HLA class I expression in post-BCG relapsed tumor (**d**). (Reprinted by permission of Wiley: Carretero et al. 2011)

response. It have been proposed that IFN-γ and epigenetically modified DFTD cells may provide a vaccine to this disease. In this context, an upregulation of HLA-I expression by interferon and MEK1/2 inhibitor selumetinib was recently reported in papillary thyroid tumors with "soft" mechanism of HLA loss (Angell et al. 2014).

In two mixed responder melanoma patients treated with autologous tumor vaccine we observed that immunotherapy can upregulate HLA I molecules and induce tumor rejection (Carretero et al. 2008). Regressing metastatic melanoma lesions after immunotherapy expressed high levels of HLA-I molecules while the progressing ones had loss HLA expression. Recovery of HLA-I expression was associated with tumor rejection, while low HLA-I expression was associated with tumor progression. In cooperation with Francesco Marincola at the NIH (USA) we did a comparative genome wide expression analysis of 15 metastasis (10 regressing and 5 progressing) obtained from these two mixed responder melanoma patients and found that the regression of melanoma metastasis is associated with an acute immune rejection mediated by the upregulation of genes involved in antigen presentation and interferon mediated response (RF-1) in all the regressing metastasis from both patients. In contrast, progressing metastasis showed low transcription levels of genes involved in these pathways. Out of the 30.000 genes analyzed only 146 genes were differentially expressed, most of which were involved in immune functions, including HLA and IFN genes (Carretero et al. 2012). The molecular signature obtained in melanoma rejection seems to be similar to that observed in other forms of immune-mediated tissue-specific rejection, such as allograft rejection, pathogen clearance, graf versus host reaction or autoimmune disease, suggesting an existence of a common "immunological constant of rejection" (Wang et al. 2008). Histological analysis of the metastatic melanoma lesion showed T cells and HLA-DR positive infiltrating cells in the regressing but not in the progressing metastasis (Carretero et al. 2012). We favour the idea that the major factor determining the success or failure of immunotherapy is the nature of HLA class I alteration in tumor cells (hard or soft) and not the type of immunotherapy used.

The concept of "reversible/soft" versus "irreversible/hard" molecular lesions has been recently confirmed. Zaretsky and coworkers have identified that progressing melanoma metastatic lesions obtained after immunotherapy with MoAbs against immune checkpoints molecules have mutations in the β2 microglobulin gene (a "hard" lesion). These data could explain why these patients did not respond to immunotherapy (Zaretsky et al. 2016). We obtained similar results years ago in a cooperative work with the Ludwig Institute in Brussels analyzing metastatic melanoma lesions in two patients immunized with MAGE tumor peptide MAGE-1 (Benitez et al. 1998). These patients did not respond to the therapy and we were able to demonstrate that these melanoma lesions were HLA class I negative and harbored β2 microglobulin mutations and LOH at chromosome 15. Restifo and coworkers reported in 1996 different β2 microglobulin mutations in five patients receiving immunotherapy (Restifo et al. 1996). Chang et al detected different mutations in HLA-A2 and β2m genes in melanoma cells derived from recurrent metastasis following immunotherapy (Chang et al. 2005). I believe that immunotherapy selects tumor cell harbouring "irreversible/hard" lesions, including mutations, micro or macro deletions and loss of genetic material in chromosomes harboring HLA and β2m genes, as well as alterations in the IFN signaling pathway. All these molecular defects cause failure of the immunotherapy (del Campo et al. 2012; Carretero et al. 2012; Garrido et al. 2016) (see Fig. 3.3).

As indicated before, I also propose that the newly designed cancer immunotherapies that use monoclonal antibodies against T cell regulatory molecules such as CTL4 or PDL-1, can "unblock" T cell reactivity in the tumor microenviroment and induce local release of Th type 1 cytoquines, such as IFN-α and ϒ. Now, tumor cells with "Soft" lesions can recover HLA-I expression and antigen presentation and induce T cell recogni-

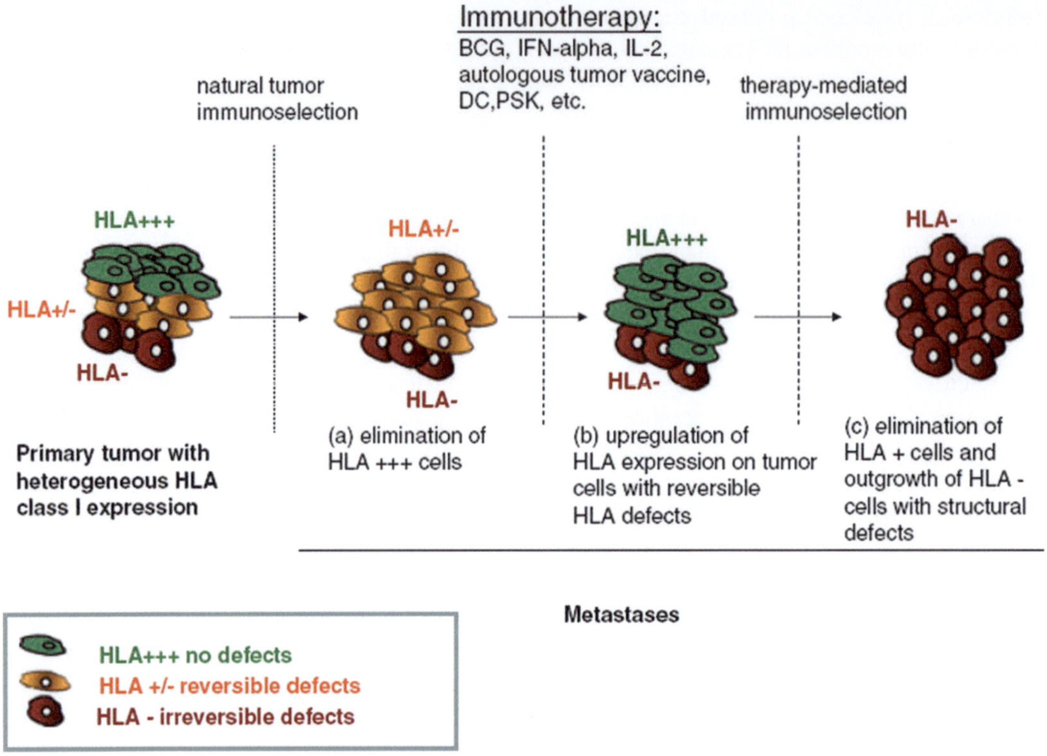

Fig. 3.3 Natural and immunotherapy-induced selection of HLA class I deficient cells harboring "hard" lesions. During natural tumor growth HLA positive tumor cells are eliminated by cytotoxic T-lymphocytes leaving behind HLA-I negative cells. They also can be eliminated by T-cells after immunotherapy (BCG, IL2, tumour peptides, dendritic cells loaded with peptides, monoclonal antibodies against T cell regulatory molecules) which can modify the tumour microenviroment and stimulate Th1 type cytoquine release. However, it can occur only in tumor cells with "reversible-soft" HLA molecular defects (green cells). However, tumor cells harbouring "irreversible-hard" molecular lesions will not recover HLA-I and will escape T-cell mediated destruction (red cells). (Reprinted by permission of Wiley: del Campo et al. 2012)

tion and tumor rejection. In contrast, tumor cells with "Hard" lesion will not recover Class I expression, will be resistant to T cell recognition and will progress (see Fig. 3.4). Indeed, resistance to checkpoint blockade therapy through inactivation of antigen presentation was recently reported and was associated with β2 microglobulin mutations and LOH (Sade-Feldman et al. 2017). These "Hard" genetic lesions were observed in tumor biopsies of seventeen metastatic melanoma patients with progressive disease. In the same study, in two independent cohorts of melanoma patients treated with anti-CTLA4 and anti PD1 respectively, LOH in β2m genetic region was enriched three-fold in responders as compared to responders and was associated with poorer overall survival.

3.2 Recovery of HLA-I Antigen Expression in Tumors with "Hard Lesions": A Challenge for the Future

Immunotherapy selects tumor cells harbouring "hard" molecular lesions that affect the antigen presentation machinery, in particular the synthesis of a functional HLA-I molecule. Loss of chromosome 6 and 15 (LOH), mutations in the β2 microglobulin and HLA-I genes and alteration in

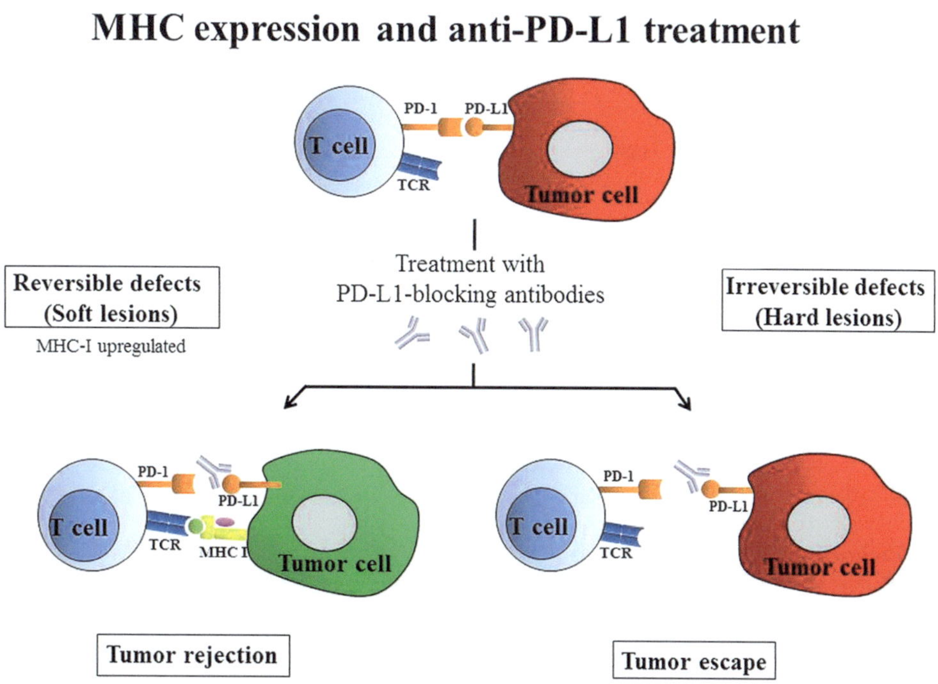

Fig. 3.4 Selection of HLA-I deficient tumor cells with "hard" lesion after anti PD-L1 treatment. Tumor cells harbouring HLA-I "soft" lesion can recover the HLA expression after treatment with anti PDL-1 treatment (green). Tumor cell with "hard" lesions do not (red)

the IFN signaling pathway have been described and represent irreversible structural alterations (Garrido et al. 2010a). The only way to recover normal tumor MHC class I expression in that case is to transfer a missing wild type gene. Indeed, soon after the first description of the loss of an H-2K^k private specificity reported in a mouse lymphoma derived from a C3H mouse (Garrido et al. 1976), several independent groups described a restoration of the expression of the missing H-2 class I specificity after an H-2 gene transfer in different tumor models, which resulted in the inhibition of tumor growth.

An AKR mouse tumor cell line K36.16 lacking K^k antigen expression was resistant to killing by AKR anti-MuLV cytotoxic lymphocytes "*in vitro*" and always produced tumors in immunocompetent syngeneic AKR mice (Festenstein et al. 1980; Festenstein and Schmidt 1981). The transfection and cell surface expression of an H-2K^k gene in the K36 (H-2K^k negative) lymphoma inhibited the syngeneic growth of this tumor (Hui et al. 1984). Similar results were obtained by Tanaka et al. in 1985 by reversing oncogenesis after transfection of the missing H-2 class I gene (Tanaka et al. 1985, 1986, 1988). Several groups did also the transfection and reexpression of the missing H-2 class I genes and molecules in (a) the B16 mouse melanoma (Wallich et al. 1985; Feldman and Eisenbach 1988), (b) in methylcholantre induced sarcomas in (C3HxC57BL/6)F1 mice (Hammerling et al. 1986) and in BALB/c mice (Mialdea et al. 1992), and (c) in Lewis lung carcinoma (Plaksin et al. 1988). These independent experiments showed similar results, namely, that the restoration of antigen presentation capacity in tumor cells harbouring H-2 class I gene losses (hard lesions) was possible and resulted in normal cell surface MHC expression leading to a recovery of T cell recognition and tumor rejection.

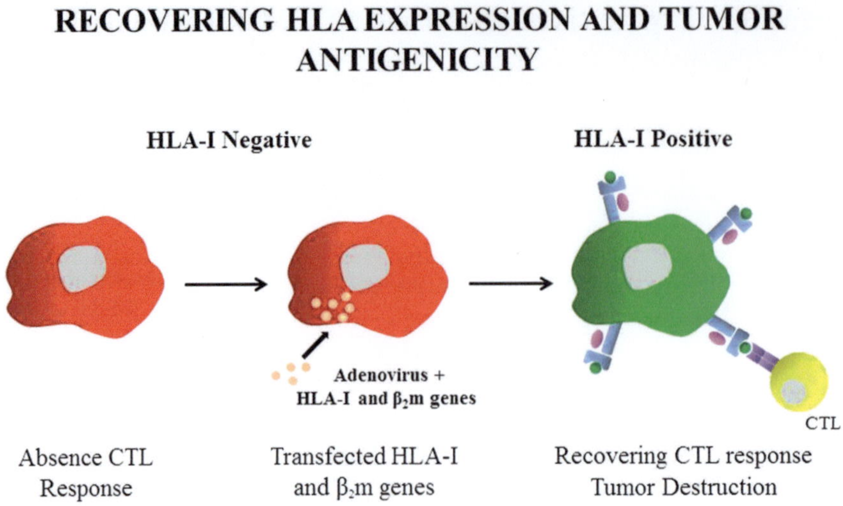

Fig. 3.5 **Recovery of HLA class I expression after the transfer of HLA-I or β2 microglobulin genes.** The transfer of class I and β2 microglobulin genes using different vectors is possible. This approach can be used in tumor cells lacking class I expression due to structural gene damage, loss of genetic material in (LOH) in chromosomes 6 and 15. The transfer leads to recovery of cell surface HLA expression and restoration of the antigen presentation capacity of the tumor cell and subsequent T cell mediated tumor recognition and elimination

We have proposed a similar approach to fight post-immunotherapy relapsed metastatic lesions harbouring irreversible "hard" lesions. Our group designed an adenoviral vector with a wild type β2m gene able to restore normal HLA class I expression in human tumor cell lines harboring β2m mutations (del Campo et al. 2009). Reconstitution of β2m expression following transduction with the adenovirus was sufficient to restore total HLA class I expression in different human tumor cells lines recovering the lysis of tumor cells by peptide-stimulated HLA-restricted T-cells and increasing peptide-specific IFN-gamma secretion by these T-cells in HLA-restricted manner (see Fig. 3.5) (del Campo et al. 2012, 2014b). We were also able to reexpress an HLA-A2 and β2 microglobulin missing genes in a particular tumor cell line with an HLA haplotype loss and a β2 microglobulin mutation indicating that it is posible to co-transfect and re-express an HLA-I missing allele together with the β2-microglobulin in a tumor cell line with both types of genetic defects (Carretero et al. 2017) (See Fig 3.6).

Different strategies have been proposed to counteract the MHC class I defects in tumors (Lampen and van Hall 2011). Attempts are in progress to revert the MHC/HLA class I tumor losses by introducing the missing element of the antigen presentation machinery (APM) or by activating transcriptional factors that regulate expression of MHC class I molecules or components of APM. NLRC5 or FHIT that recently were reported to control the transcription of class I, β2m and genes involved in antigen processing (Romero et al. 2012; Yoshihama et al. 2016). The restoration of the antigen presentation capacity in tumor cells is an urgent need in order to have an efficient cancer immunotherapy (Garrido et al. 2016). Since MHC/HLA class I

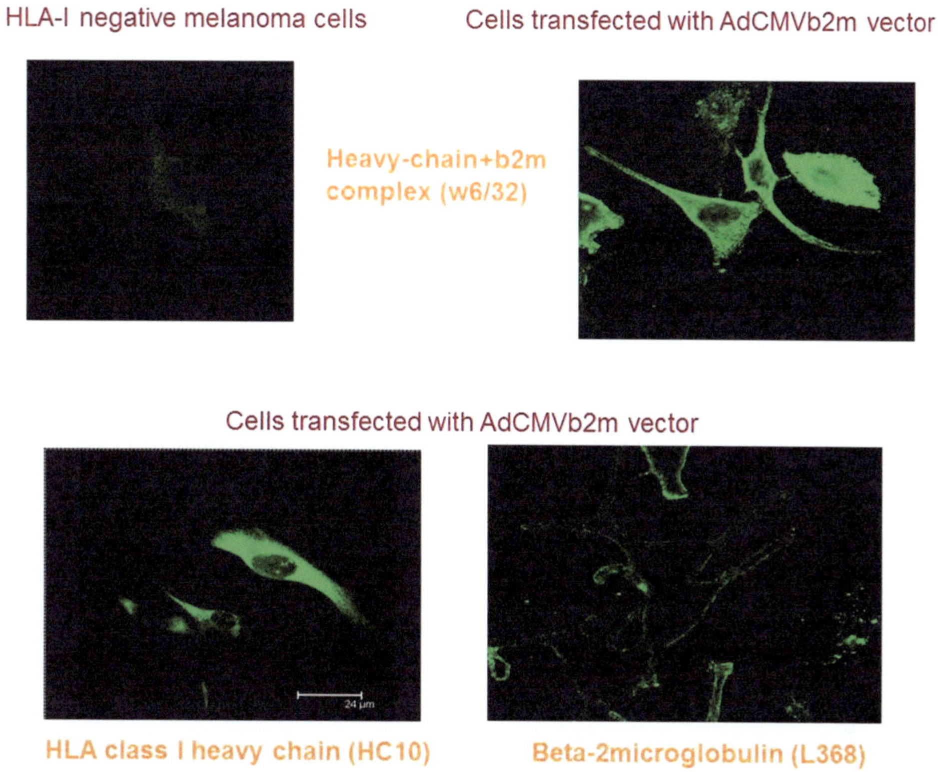

Fig. 3.6 Confocal microscopy of HLA-I negative melanoma cells transfected with an adenovirus carrying the β2 microglobulin gene. The M010 melanoma cells recover HLA class I expression after the transfer of the wild-type β2m gene. MOLO cells are deficient in β2m genes due to a point mutation and LOH in chromosome 15 (del Campo et al. 2014a, b). We used MoAbs against a common HLA-ABC determinant (w6/32), against the free intracytoplasmic HLA heavy chain and against β2 microglobulin

losses can be produced by a variety of molecular mechanisms, it will be necessary to define strategies to precisely diagnose in each tumor what particular approach need be used. In this context, we have defined predictable patterns of HLA-I molecular alterations that happens in different tumors in order to help choosing strategies to perform a quick HLA analysis in tumor tissues (Cabrera et al. 2007).

References

Abril E, Real LM, Serrano A, Jimenez P, Garcia A, Canton J, Trigo I, Garrido F, Ruiz-Cabello F (1998) Unresponsiveness to interferon associated with STAT1 protein deficiency in a gastric adenocarcinoma cell line. Cancer Immunol Immunother 47:113–120

Andersen R, Donia M, Ellebaek E, Holz Borch T, Kongsted P, Iversen TZ, Rosenkrantz Hölmich L, Westergren Hendel H, Met O, Hald AM, Thor Straten P, Svane IM

(2016) Long-lasting complete responses in patients with metastatic melanoma after adoptive cell therapy with tumor-infiltrating lymphocytes and an attenuated IL-2 regimen. Clin Cancer Res 22(15):3734–3745

Angell TE, Lechner MG, Jang JK, LoPresti JS, Epstein AL (2014) MHC class I loss is a frequent mechanism of immune escape in papillary thyroid cancer that is reversed by interferon and selumetinib treatment in vitro. Clin Cancer Res 20:6034–6044

Aptsiauri N, Carretero R, Garcia-Lora A, Real LM, Cabrera T, Garrido F (2008) Regressing and progressing metastatic lesions: Resistance to immunotherapy is predetermined by irreversible HLA class I antigen alterations. Cancer Immunol Immunother 57:1727–1733

Aptsiauri N, Garcia-Lora A, Garrido F (2014) Chapter 5: "Hard" and "Soft" loss of MHC class I expression in cancer cells. In: Rees B (ed) Tumour immunology & immunotherapy. Oxford University Press, pp 63–78

Benitez R, Godelaine D, Lopez-Nevot MA, Brasseur F, Jimenez P, Marchand M, Oliva MR, van Baren N, Cabrera T, Andry G, Landry C, Ruiz-Cabello F, Boon T, Garrido F (1998) Mutations of the β2-microglobulin gene result in a lack of HLA class I molecules on melanoma cells of two patients immunized with MAGE peptides. Tissue Antigens 52:520–529

Bernal M, Ruiz-Cabello F, Concha A, Paschen A, Garrido F (2012) Implication of the β2 microglobuline gene in the generation of tumour escape phenotypes. Cancer Immunol Immunother 61(9):1359–1371

Cabrera T, Maleno I, Collado A, Lopez-Nevot MA, Tait B, Garrido F (2007) Analysis of HLA class I alterations in tumours: choosing a strategy based on known patterns of underlying molecular mechanisms. Tissue Antigens 69(Suppl 1):264–268

Carretero R, Romero JM, Ruiz-Cabello F, Maleno I, Rodriguez F, Camacho FM, Real LM, Garrido F, Cabrera T (2008) Analysis of HLA class I expression in progressing and regressing metastatic melanoma lesions after immunotherapy. Immunogenetics 60:439–447

Carretero R, Cabrera T, Sáenz-López P, Maleno I, Aptsiauri N, Cózar JM, Garrido F (2011) Bacillus Calmette-Guerin immunotherapy of bladder cancer induces selection of human leukocyte antigen class I-deficient tumor cells. Int J Cancer 129(4):839–846

Carretero R, Wang E, Rodriguez AI, Reinboth J, Ascierto ML, Engle AM, Liu H, Camacho F, Marincola FM, Garrido F, Cabrera T (2012) Regression of melanoma metastases after immunotherapy is associated with activation of antigen presentation and interferon-mediated rejection genes. Int J Cancer 131:387–395

Carretero FJ, Del Campo AB, Zinchenko S, Garrido F, Aptsiauri N (2017) Recovery HLA-A2 and β2-microglobulin expression in tumor cells using viral vectors. J Cancer Sci Ther 9:622–629

Chang CC, Campoli M, Restifo NP, Wang X, Ferrone S (2005) Immune selection of hot-spot β2 microglobuline gene mutations, HLA-A2 alloespecificity loss and antigen processing machinery component downregulation in melanoma cells derived from recurrent metastasis following immunotherapy. J Immunol 174:1462–1471

del Campo AB, Aptsiauri N, Méndez R, Zinchenko S, Vales A, Paschen A, Ward S, Ruiz-Cabello F, González-Aseguinolaza G, Garrido F (2009) Efficient recovery of HLA class I expression in human tumor cells after β2-microglobulin gene transfer using adenoviral vector: implicationsfor cancer immunotherapy. Scand J Immunol 70(2):125–135

del Campo AB, Carretero J, Aptsiauri N, Garrido F (2012) Targeting HLA class I expression to increase tumor immunogenicity. Tissue Antigens 79(3):147–154

del Campo AB, Kyte JA, Carretero J, Zinchencko S, Mendez R, Gonzalez-Aseguinolaza G, Ruiz-Cabello F, Aamdal S, Gaudernac G, Garrido F, Aptsiauri N (2014a) Immune escape of cancer cells with β2 microglobuline loss over the course of metastatic melanoma. Int J Cancer 134(1):102–113

del Campo AB, Carretero J, Muñoz JA, Zinchenko S, Ruiz-Cabello, Gonzalez-Aseguinolaza G, Garrido F, Aptsiauri N (2014b) Adenovirus expressing β2 microglobuline recovers HLA class I expression and antitumor immunity by increasing T cell recognition. Cancer Gene Ther 21(8):317–332

Feldman M, Eisenbach L (1988) Genes controlling the metastatic phenotype. Cancer Surv 7:555–572

Festenstein, Schmidt W (1981) Variation in MHC antigen profile of tumour cells and its biological effect. Immunol Rev 60:85

Festenstein H, Schmidt W, Testorelli C, Marelli O, Simpson S (1980) Biologic effects of the altered MHS profile on the K36 tumor, a spontaneous leukemia of AKR. Transplant Proc 12(1):25–28

Garrido F, Festenstein H, Schirrmacher V (1976) Further evidence for derepression of H-2 and Ia-likespecificities of foreign haplotypes in mouse tumour cell lines. Nature 261(5562):705–707

Garrido F, Cabrera T, Aptsiauri N (2010a) "Hard" and "Soft" lesions underlying the HLA class I alterations in cancer cells: implications for immunotherapy. Int J Cancer 127(2):249–256

Garrido F, Algarra I, García-Lora AM (2010b) The escape of cancer from T lymphocytes: immunoselection of MHC class I loss variants harboring structural-irreversible "hard" lesions. Cancer Immunol Immunother 59(10):1601–1606

Garrido C, Romero I, Berruguilla E, Cancela B, Algarra I, Collado A, Garcia-Lora AM, Garrido F (2011) Immunotherapy eradicates metastases with reversible defects in MHC class I expression. Cancer Immunol Immunother 60(9):1257–1268

Garrido F, Aptsiauri N, Doorduijn E, Garcia-Lora A, van Hall T (2016) The urgent need to recover MHC class I in cancers for effective immunotherapy. Curr Opin Immunol 39:44–51

Garrido G, Rabasa A, Garrido C, Lisset C, Garrido F, Garcia-Lora A, Sanchez-Ramirez B (2017) Upregulation of HLA class I expression on tumour cells by the anti-EGFR antibody Nimotuzumab. Front Pharmacol. https://doi.org/10.3389/fphar.2017.00595

Hammerling G, Klar D, Katzav S, Segal S, Feldman M, Wallich R, Hammerling A (1986) Manipulation of metastasis and tumor growth by transfection with histocompatibility class I genes. J Immunogenet 13:153–157

Hui K, Grosveld F, Festenstein H (1984) Rejection of transplantable AKR leukaemia cells following MHC DNA-mediated cell transformation. Nature 311(5988):750–752

Kloor M, Michel S, von Knebel Doeberitz M (2010) Immune evasion of microsatelite unstable colorectal cancers. Int J Cancer 127:1001–1010

Lampen MH, van Hall T (2011) Strategies to counteract MHC-I defects in tumors. Curr Opin Immunol 23:293–298

Leach MF, Krummel DR, Allison JP (1996) Enhancement of anti tumour immunity by CTL-4 blockade. Science 271(5256):1734–1736

Maleno I, Romero JM, Cabrera T, Paco L, Aptsiauri N, Cozar JM, Tallada M, Lopez-Nevot MA, Garrido F (2006) LOH at 6p21.3 region and HLA class I altered phenotypes in bladder carcinomas. Immunogenetics 58:503–510

Maleno I, Aptsiauri N, Cabrera T, Gallego A, Paschen A, Lopez- Nevot MA, Garrido F (2011) Frequent loss of heterozygosity in the β2-microglobulin region of chromosome 15 in primary human tumors. Immunogenetics 63:65–71

Marchand M, Weynants P, Rankin E, Arienti F, Belli F, Parmiani G, Cascinelli N, Bourlond A, Vanwijch R, Humblet et al (1995) Tumour regression responses in melanoma patients treated with a peptide encoded by gene MAGE-3. Int J Cancer 63:883–889

Marchand M, Van Baren N, Weynan P, Brichard V, Dreno B, Tessier M-H, Rankin E, Parmiani G, Arienti F, Humblet Y, Bourlond A, Vanwijck R, Lienard D, Beauduin M, Dietrich P-Y, Russo V, Kerger J, Masucci G, Jager E, De Greve J, Atzpodien J, Brasseur F, Coulie P, Van Der Bruggen P, Boon T (1999) Tumour regressions observed in patients with metastatic melanoma treated with an antigenic peptide encoded by gene MAGE-3 and presented by HLA-A1. Int J Cancer 89:219–230

Mendez R, Ruiz-Cabello F, Jimenez P, Paschen A, Knuth A, Jager E, Traversari C, Schadendorf D, Boon T, Garrido F (2006) Impact of HLA class I alterations in patients undergoing T cell specific immunotherapy. Immunobiology of the human MHC. In: Proceedings of the 13th International Histocompatibility Workshop and Conference (IHWC) 2002, vol 2, IHWG Press, pp 512–514

Mialdea MJ, Martin J, Gaforio JJ, Algarra I, Perez M, Gonzalez A, Ljunggren HG, Garrido F (1992) Effect of MHC class I transfection on local tumour growth and metastasis in an H-2 negative clone derived from a chemically induced fibrosarcoma. Int J Cancer 52:153–158

Morales A, Eidinger D, Bruce AW (1976) Intracavitary Bacillus Calmette Guerin in the treatment of superficial bladder tumors. J Urol 116:180–183

Nestle FO, Alijagic S, Gilliet M, Sun Y, Grabbe S, Dummer R, Burg G, Shadendorf D (1998) Vaccination of melanoma patients with peptide or tumor lysate-pulsed dendritic cells. Nature (Med) 4:328–332

Nio Y, Shiraishi T, Tsubono M, Morimoto H, Tseng C Imai S, Tobe T (1991) In vitro immunomodulating effect of protein-bound polysaccharide,PSK on peripheral blood, regional nodes and spleen lymphocytes in patients with gastric cancer. Cancer Immunol Immunother 32:335–339

Plaksin D, Gelber C, Feldman M, Eisenbach L (1988) Reversal of the metastatic phenotype in Lewis lung carcinoma cells after transfection with syngeneic H-$2K^b$ gene. Proc Natl Acad Sci U S A 85(12):4463–4467

Porgador A, Brenner E, Vadai M, Feldman M, Eisenbach L (1991) Immunization by gamma-IFN-treated B16-F10.9 melanoma cells protects against metastatic spread of the parental tumor. Int J Cancer Suppl 6:54–60

Restifo NP, Marincola FM, Kawakami Y, Taubenberger J, Yanelli JR, Rosenberg SA (1996) Loss of functional β2-microglobulin in metastatic melanoma from five patients receiving immunotherapy. J Natl Cancer Inst 88:100–108

Rodriguez T, Mendez R, Del Campo A, Jimenez P, Aptsiauri N, Garrido F, Ruiz-Cabello F (2007) Distinct mechanisms of loss of IFN-gamma mediated HLA class I inducibility in two melanoma cell lines. BMC Cancer 7:34

Romero I, Martinez M, Garrido C, Collado A, Algarra I, Garrido F, Garcia-Lora AM (2012) The tumour suppressor Fhit positively regulates MHC class I expression on cancer cells. J Pathol 227(3):367–379

Rosenberg SA, Lotze MT, Muul LM (1987) A progress report on the treatment of 157 patients with advance cáncer using lymphokine-activated killer cells and interleukin-2 or high-dose interleukin-2 alone. N Engl J Med 316(15):889–897

Ruiz-Cabello F, Garrido F (1998) HLA and cancer: from research to clinical impact. Immunol Today 19:539–542

Ruiz-Cabello F, Cabrera T, Lopez-Nevot MA, Garrido F (2002) Impaired surface antigen presentation in tumors: implications for T cell-based immunotherapy. Semin Cancer Biol 12:15–24

Sade-Feldman M, Jiao Y, Chen J, Rooney M, Barzily-Rokni M, Eliane JP, Bjorgaard S, Hammond M, Vitzthum H, Blackmon S et al (2017) Resistance to checkpoint blockade therapy throught inactivation of antigen presentation. Nat Commun 8:1136. https://doi.org/10.1038/s41467-017-01062

Seliger B, Ruiz-Cabello F, Garrido F (2008) IFN inducibility of major histocompatibility antigens in tumors. Adv Cancer Res 101:249–276

Sharma P, Allison JP (2015) The future of immune checkpoint therapy. Science 348(6230):56–61

Siddle HV, Kreiss A, Tovar C, Yuen CK, Chang Y, Belov K, Swift K, Pearse AM, Hamede R, Jones ME, Skjodt K, Woods GM, Kaufman J (2013) Reversible epigenetic down-regulation of MHC molecules by devil facial tumour disease illustrate immune escape by a contagious cancer. Proc Natl Acad Sci U S A 110(13):5103–5108

Sucker A, Zhao F, Pieper N, Heeke C, Maltaner R, Stadtler N, Real B, Bielefeld N, Howe S, Weide B, Gutzmer R, Utikal J, Loquai C, Gogas H, Klein-Hitpass L, Zeschnigk M, Westendorf A, Trilling M, Horn S, Schilling B, Schadendorf D, Griewank K, Paschen A (2017) Adquired IFNγ resistance impairs anti-tumor immunity and gives rise to T-cell-resistance melanoma lesions. Nat Commun 31(8):15440. https://doi.org/10.1038/ncomms15440

Tanaka K, Isselbacher KJ, Khoury G, Jay G (1985) Reversal of oncogenesis by the expression of major histocompatibility complex class I gene. Science 228:26–30

Tanaka K, Hayashi H, Hamada C, Khoury G, Jay G (1986) Expression of major histocompatibility complex class-I antigens as a strategy for the potentiation of immune recognition of tumor cells. Proc Natl Acad Sci (Was) 83:8723–8727

Tanaka K, Gorelik E, Watanabe M, Hozumi N, Jay G (1988) Rejection of B16 melanoma induced by expression of a transfected major histocompatibility complex class-I gene. Mol Cell Biol 8:1857–1861

Thor Straten P, Garrido F (2016) Targetless T cells in cancer immunotherapy. J Immunother Cancer 19(4):23–26

Tsukagoshi S, Hashimoto Y, Fujii G, Kobayashi H, Nomoto K, Orita K (1984) PSK. Cancer Treat Rew 11:131–139

Wallich R, Bulbuc N, Hammerling GJ, Katzav S, Segal S, Feldman M (1985) Abrogation of metastasis properties of tumor cells by de novo expression of H-2K antigens following H-2 gene transfection. Nature 315:301–307

Wang E, Worschech A, Marincola FM (2008) The immunological constant of rejection. Trends Immunol 29:256–262

Woods GM, Howson LJ, Brown GK, Tovar C, Kreiss A, Corcoran LM, Lyons AB (2015) Immunology of a transmissible cancer spreading among Tasmanian Devils. J Immunol 195:23–29

Yoshihama S, Roszik J, Downs I, Meissner T, Vijayan S, Chapuy B, Sidiq T, Shipp M, Lizee G, Kobayashi K (2016) NLRC5/MHC class I transactivator is a target for immune evasión in cancer. PNAS 113:5999–6004

Zaretsky JM, Garcia-Diaz A, Shin DS, Escuin-Ordinas H, Hugo W, Hu-Lieskovan S, Torrejon DY, Abril-Rodriguez G, Sandoval S, Barthly et al (2016) Mutations associated with acquired resistance to PD-1 blockade in melanoma. N Engl J Med 375:819–829

HLA Class-II Expression in Human Tumors

4

Abstract
HLA class II molecules play a pivotal role in antigen presentation to T lymphocytes. This chapter analyzed the expression of these molecules in different human tumors and their role in cancer progression. The possible connection between tumor HLA class II expression and the pathogenesis of autoimmune diseases is discussed.

Keywords
HLA-II in tissues · HLA-II in tumors · Antigen presenting cells · Interferon · Tumor rejection · Tumor prognosis · HLA-II & autoimmunity · Immunohistochemistry · Tumor infiltrating lymphocytes · Cytokynes

HLA class II molecules (HLA-DR, DP and DQ) are rectricted in their tissue distribution in human tissues. Normally they are expressed in antigen presenting cells of the immune system, including dendritic and Langherhan cells, monocytes, macrophages and B lymphocytes. Activated T lymphocytes also express class II molecules. They have a constitutive expression but also can be strongly induced by different cytoquines including IFN and TNF. They are known to play a major role in presenting antigens to CD4 positive lymphocytes. Extracelullar antigens coming mostly from bacteria are processed by Antigen-Presenting Cells (APCs) that are very rich in HLA-II expression and can induce humoral immune responses.

Early reports showed that HLA class II antigens are expressed in different tissues of the gastrointestinal tract (tongue, duodenum, ileum), respiratory system (epiglottis, traquea), urogenital system (glomeruli, tubules, urethra) (Natali et al. 1981; Daar et al. 1984). For details see table I in chapter I. Normal melanocytes unlike Langerghans cells do not express HLA class II antigens when studied by immunohistochemistry (van Duinen et al. 1984). We have found that epithelial cells of the colon (Gutierrez et al. 1987), larynx (Esteban et al. 1990), skin (Cabrera et al. 1992), muscle and squamous and columnar ephitelium cells of the cervix (Glew et al. 1992) do not express HLA-DR antigens. In contrast, weak HLA-DR antigen expression was observed in stomach (Ferron et al. 1989), lung (Redondo et al. 1991) and breast parenquima (Concha et al. 1995). It is interesting to note that epithelia that are affected by external stimuli can be either HLA-DR positive (lung and stomach) or HLA-DR negative (colon, larynx, cervix and skin).

Expression of MHC class II in tumors was first reported on human melanoma cell lines by Wilson et al. (1979). Displastic nevi show local expression of HLA class II in about 20% of the lesions (Ruiter et al. 1982; D'Alessandro et al. 1987). HLA class II expression has been reported in 40–70% of primary cutaneous melanomas (Ruiter

F. Garrido, *MHC Class-I Loss and Cancer Immune Escape*, Advances in Experimental Medicine and Biology 1151, https://doi.org/10.1007/978-3-030-17864-2_4

et al. 1984; Zaloudik et al. 1988). The frequency of HLA class II expression in melanoma metastases depends on the stage of the lesion and has been reported in around 80% of loco-regional metastases and only in 10% of distant cutaneous metastases. Different publications indicate that HLA class II antigens are expressed in a subpopulation of human tumors (Daar et al. 1982; Moore et al. 1986; Gutierrez et al. 1987; Garrido et al. 1993; Cabrera et al. 1995). For instance, HLA DR, DP and DQ are differentially expressed in colon adenomas and in carcinomas (Degener et al. 1998) and HLA DR was detected in a subpopulation of colorectal cancer (Daar et al. 1982; Ghosh et al. 1986). Gutierrez et al showed that normal colon mucosa is HLA class II negative except in mucosa adjacent to the tumor and in polyp adenomas the intensity was paralleled by the degree of dysplasia (Gutierrez et al. 1987). In this same study, HLA-DR was detected in 50% of carcinomas with no relationship with the degree of differentiation, however, tumors with more favourable prognosis (stages I–II) were HLA-DR positive while those with the worst prognosis (stages III–IV) were HLA-DR negative. Interestingly, HLA class II antigen expression in "familial polyposis coli" is related to the degree of dysplasia implying that is somehow related with malignant transformation (Gutierrez et al. 1990).

The biological significance of such findings is still unclear. For instance, HLA-DR molecules are expressed in 12% of laryngeal carcinomas and are associated with low grade of tumor differentiation and excellent prognosis (Esteban et al. 1990). Similarly, Andersen and coworkers reported that HLA-DR expression in large bowel carcinomas is associated with good prognosis (Andersen et al. 1993). Concha et al. (1991), Natali et al. (1983) and Brunner et al. (1991) reported that HLA class II is associated with good prognosis in breast carcinomas. Constitutive expression of HLA-DR antigens in high-degree B cell lymphomas has been associated with less aggressive behavior in these neoplasms (Momburg et al. 1987; Spier et al. 1988). In contrast, HLA-DR expression in melanoma was associated with a poor prognosis since it was detected in a high proportion of metastasis (Brocker et al. 1985; Lopez-Nevot et al. 1986, 1988; Taramelli et al. 1986). I recommend reading the review written by Cabrera and coworkers that summarizes the biological implications of HLA-DR expression in tumors (Cabrera et al. 1995).

The expression of HLA-DR in tissues is also playing an important role in the induction of autoimmune diseases as was described in autoimmune thyroiditis (Jansson et al. 1984) and autoimmune induced type-I diabetes (Botazzo et al. 1985). HLA class II expression also is involved in the pathogenesis of celiac disease which is known to be linked with the wheat derived gluten intolerance (Stamnaes and Sollid 2015). Gluten is highly abundant in the modern diet and well tolerated by most individuals. In celiac disease, an erroneous but highly specific adaptive immune response is mounted toward certain parts of the gluten proteome. Post-translational modification (deamination) of gluten peptides by transglutaminase-2 is essential for peptides to act as HLA-DQ-restricted T cell antigens. The presence of an inherited particular HLA-DQ2 allele is responsible for the processing of a particular peptided derived from a transglutaminase in the colorectal epithelia raising a T cell mediated immune response (Lundin and Sollid 2014). An HLA-DQ-Gluten tetramer blood test has been recently set up that accurately identifies patients with and without celiac disease in absence of gluten consumption (Sarna et al. 2018).These data emphazise the existing association between HLA class II expression in autoimmune disease and cancer because of its role in antigen presentation. It is also possible to hypothesize that HLA class II expression might have two opposite effects, a positive contribution in case of tumours with good prognosis and a harmful one in autoimmune diseases with increased tissue damage (Cabrera et al. 1995). These ideas fit with the concept that there is an "immunological constant of rejection" of both autoimmune reactivity and immune reactions aimed at tumor destruction (Wang et al. 2008).

We have recently observed in lung and colorectal cancer tissues that HLA DR expression is associated with T lymphocyte infiltration in "HLA-class I negative tumors" suggesting that

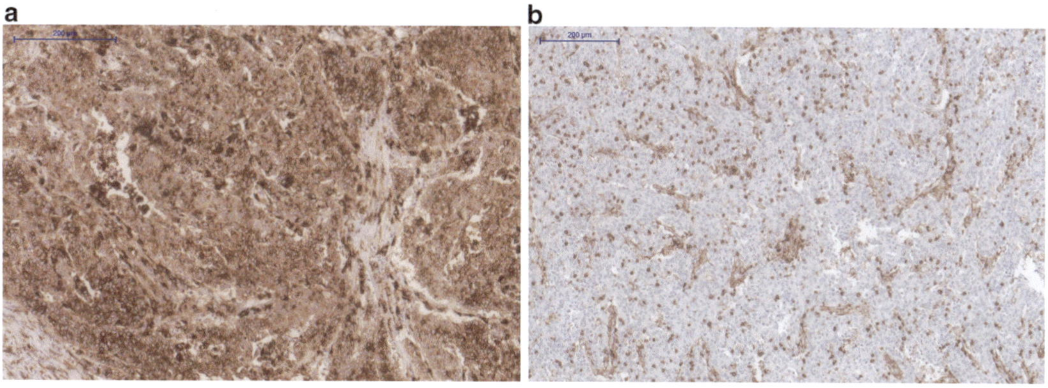

Fig. 4.1 Expression of class II is associated with high leucocyte infiltration in an HLA class I negative CRC. MSH-I Colorectal carcinoma is HLA class II homogeneously positive (**a**) Is heavily infiltrated with CD45 positive cells within the tumor nests (**b**)

HLA class II expression might be playing an important role in tumor rejection when the escape route via HLA-I is already established (Perea et al. 2018) See Fig. 4.1. The absence of HLA class II molecules in tumors is sometimes caused by mutations in HLA class II regulatory genes (Michel et al. 2010) but it can also be inducible with different cytokines including IFNs indicating that also "reversible/soft" and irreversible/hard" molecular mechanisms are also detected in HLA class II abnormalities. The analysis of HLA-II expression in tumors that lack HLA-I molecules is an important area of research for future studies. Finally, it is also useful to remember that there is a congenital immunodeficiency disease known as "Bare lymphocyte syndrome" that is characterized by the absence of mRNA specific for class II molecules despite the presence of intact HLA class II genes that cannot be activated by γ-IFN. The absence of a transcription factor (RF-X) in B lymphocytes is thought to be responsible for this defect (Stimac et al. 1991; Hasegawa et al. 1993).

Future studies of HLA class II in tumors will need to take into account the differential expression of HLA- DR, DQ and DP molecules in tumor tissues and the role that each of these different locus products play in tumor rejection. We analyzed forty two melanoma cell lines from the European Searchable Tumour cell line data base (ESTDAB project, http://www.ebi.ac.uk/ipd/estdab) for HLA class II expression by flow cytometry before and after IFN treatment (Rodriguez et al. 2007; Pawelec and Marsh 2006). The results showed that twenty four cell lines were class II negative for the three locus products but could induce DR and DP in 50% of the cases. Interestingly, only one cell line out of the twenty four recovered HLA-DQ expression. The constitutive positive expression of HLA-DR and DQ was similar in sixteen cell lines, while HLA-DQ was negative in ten cell lines, although it could be recovered after IFN treatment only in two cases (Rodriguez et al. 2007).

The biological implications of HLA class II expression in tumor cells and CD4+ T cell infiltration in tumor tissues has been investigated for the past years (Ostrand-Rosenberg 2005), but, nevertheless, it needs more detailed analysis. It can be hypothesized that in some types of tumors this expression gives tumor cells the ability to present antigens to become less aggressive with overall better prognosis. In vitro transfection assays in a melanoma showed that HLA class II positive cells were able to function as antigen presenting cells (Chen et al. 1994) and MHC class II transfectans obtained in a variety of mouse tumors were very effective vaccines against subsequent challenge with wild type class II tumors (Ostrand-Rosenberg et al. 1990). HLA-II expression can be also a marker of tumor differentiation and it is well established that it can be also induced by locally released cytokines in the tumor microenviroment.

References

Andersen SN, Rognum TO, Lund E, Meling GI, Hauge S (1993) Strong HLA-DR expression in large bowel carcinomas is associated with good prognosis. Br J Cancer 68:80–85

Botazzo F, Dean BM, McNally JM, MacKay EH, Swift PG, Gamble DR (1985) In situ characterization of autoimmune phenomena and expression of HLA molecules in the pancreas in diabetes insulitis. N Engl J Med 313(6):353–360

Brocker EB, Suter L, Bruggen J, Ruiter DJ, Macher E, Sorg C (1985) Phenotypic dinamics of tumour progression in human malignant melanoma. Int J Cancer 36:29–35

Brunner CA, Gokel JM, Riethmuller G, Johnson JP (1991) Expression of HLA-D subloci DR and DQ by breast carcinomas is correlated with distinct parameters of favourable prognosis. Eur J Cancer 27:411–416

Cabrera T, Garrido V, Concha A, Martin J, Esquivias J, Oliva MR, Ruiz-Cabello F, Serrano S, Garrido F (1992) HLA molecules in basal cell carcinoma of the skin. Immunobiology 185:440–452

Cabrera T, Ruiz-Cabello F, Garrido F (1995) Biological implications of HLA-DR expression in tumours. Scand J Immunol 41:398–406

Chen P, Ullrich S, Ananthaswamy H (1994) Presentation of endogenous tumor antigens to CD4+ T lymphocytes by murine melanoma cells transfected with major histocompatibility complex class II genes. J Leukocyte Biol 56:469–474

Concha A, Esteban F, Cabrera T, Ruiz-Cabello F, Garrido F (1991) Tumor aggressiveness and MHC class I and II antigens in laryngeal and breast cancer. Semin Cancer Biol 2:47–54

Concha A, Ruiz-Cabello F, Cabrera T, Nogales F, Collado A, Garrido F (1995) Different patterns of HLA-DR antigen expression in normal epithelium, hyperplastic and neoplastic malignant lesions of the breast. Eur J Immunogenet 22:299–310

D'Alessandro G, Zardawi I, Grace J, McCarthy WH, Hersey P (1987) Immunohistological evaluation of MHC class I and II antigen expression on nevi and melanoma: relation to biology of melanoma. Pathology 19:339–346

Daar AS, Fuggle SV, Ting A, Fabre JW (1982) Anomalous expression of HLA DR antigens on human colorectal cancer cells. J Immunol 129:447

Daar AS, Fuggle SV, Fabre JW, Ting A, Morris P (1984) The detail distribution of MHC class II antigens in normal human organs. Transplantation 38:293–298

Degener T, Momburg F, Moller P (1998) Differential expression of HLA-DR, HLA-DP, HLA-DQ and associated invariant chain (II) in normal colorectal mucosa, adenoma and carcinoma. Virchows Arch A 412:315–322

Esteban F, Ruiz-Cabello F, Concha A, Perez-Ayala M, Sanchez-Rozas JA, Garrido F (1990) HLA-DR expression is associated with excellent prognosis in squamous cell carcinoma of the larynx. Clin Exp Metastasis 8:319–328

Ferron A, Perez-Ayala M, Concha A, Cabrera T, Redondo M, Oliva MR, Ruiz-Cabello F, Garrido F (1989) MHC class I and II antigens on gastric carcinomas and autologous mucosa. J Immunogenet 16:413–423

Garrido F, Cabrera T, Concha A, Glew S, Ruiz-Cabello F, Stern PL (1993) Natural history of HLA expression during tumour development. Immunol Today 14:491–499

Ghosh AK, Moore M, Street AJ, Howat JMT, Schofield PF (1986) Expression of HLA-D subregion products on human colorectal carcinoma. Int J Cancer 38:459–464

Glew SS, Duggan-Keen M, Cabrera T, Stern P (1992) HLA class II antigen expression in human papillomavirus associated cervical cancer. Cancer Res 52:1–8

Gutierrez J, Lopez-Nevot MA, Cabrera T, Oliva R, Esquivias J, Ruiz-Cabello F, Garrido F (1987) Class I ans II HLA antigen distribution in normal mucosa, adenoma and colon carcinoma: relation with malignancy and invasiveness. Exp Clin Immunogenet 4:144–152

Gutierrez J, Ruiz-Cabello F, Lopez-Nevot MA, Cabrera T, Esquivias J, Garrido F (1990) Class II HLA antigen expression in familial polyposis coli is related to the degree of dysplasia. Immunobiology 180:138–148

Hasegawa SL, James LR, Sloan JH, Boos JM (1993) Protease treatment of nuclear extracts distinguishes between class II major histocompatibility complex X1 box DNA-binding proteins in wild type and class II deficient B cells. J Immunol 150:1781–1793

Jansson R, Karlsson A, Forsum U (1984) Intrathyroidal HLA-DR expression and T lymphocyte phenotypes in Graves's thyrotoxicosis, Hasimoto's thyroiditis and nodular colloid goitre. Clin Exp Immunol 58:264–272

Lopez-Nevot MA, Garcia E, Pareja E, Bonal E, Martin F, Ruiz-Cabello F, Serrano S, Garrido F (1986) Differential expression of HLA class I and II antigens in primary and metastatic melanomas. J Immunogenet 13(2/3):219–228

Lopez-Nevot MA, Garcia E, Romero C, Oliva MR, Serrano S, Garrido F (1988) Phenotypic and genetic analysis of HLA class I and HLA-DR antigen expression on human melanomas. Exp Clin Immunogenet 5:203–212

Lundin K, Sollid L (2014) Advances in celiac disease. Curr Opin Gastroenterol 30(2):154–162

Michel S, Linnebacher M, Alcañiz J, Voss M, Wagner R, Dippold W, Becker C, von Knebel Doeberitz M, Ferrone M, Kloor M (2010) Lack of HLA class II antigen expression in microsatellite unstable colorectal carcinomas is caused by mutations in HLA class II regulatory genes. Int J Cancer 127(4):889–898

Momburg F, Herrmann B, Moldehauer G, Moller PB (1987) B cell lymphomas of high-grade malignancy frequently lack HLA-DR, DP and DQ antigens and associated invariant chain. Int J Cancer 40:598–603

Moore M, Ghosh D, Johnston D, Street J (1986) Expression of MHC class II products on human

colorectal cancer: an immunohistological and flow cytometric study. J Immunogenet 13:201–209
Natali PG, De Martino C, Quaranta V, Nicotra MR, Frezza F, Pellegrino MA, Ferrone S (1981) Expression of Ia like antigens in normal human non-lymphoid tissues. Transplantation 31:75–78
Natali PG, Giacomini P, Bigotti A, Imai K, Nicotra MR, Ferrone S (1983) Heterogeneity in the expression of HLA and tumor associated antigens by surgically removed and cultured breast carcinoma cells. Cancer Res 43:660–668
Ostrand-Rosenberg S (2005) CD4+ T lymphocytes: a critical component of antitumor immunity. Cancer Invest 23:413–419
Ostrand-Rosenberg S, Thakur A, Clements V (1990) Rejection of mouse sarcoma cells after transfection of MHC-class II genes. J Immunol 144:4068–4071
Pawelec G, Marsh SG (2006) ESTDAB: a collection of immunologically characterized melanoma cell lines and searchable databank. Cancer Immunol Immunother 55:623–627
Perea F, Sánchez-Palencia A, Gómez-Morales M, Bernal M, Concha Á, García MM, González-Ramírez AR, Kerick M, Martin J, Garrido F, Ruiz-Cabello F, Aptsiauri N (2018) HLA class I loss and PD-L1 expression in lung cancer: impact on T-cell infiltration and immune escape. Oncotarget 9(3):4120–4133. https://doi.org/10.18632/oncotarget.23469. eCollection 2018 Jan 9. PubMed PMID: 29423109; PubMed Central PMCID: PMC5790526
Redondo M, Concha A, Oldiviela R, Cueto A, Gonzalez A, Garrido F, Ruiz-Cabello (1991) Expression of HLA class I and II antigens in bronchogenic carcinomas: its relationship to cellular DNA content and clinic-pathological parameters. Cancer Res 51:4948–4954
Rodriguez T, Mendez R, De Campo A, Aptsiauri N, Martin J, Orozco G, Pawelec G, Shadendorf D, Ruiz-Cabello F, Garrido F (2007) Patterns of constitutive and IFN-γ inducible expression of HLA class II molecules in human melanoma cell lines. Immunogenetics 59:123–133
Ruiter DJ, Bhan AK, Harrist TJ, Sober AJ, Mihm MC (1982) Major histocompatibility antigens and mononuclear inflammatory infiltrate in benign nevomelanocytic proliferations and malignant melanoma. J Immunol 129:2808–2815
Ruiter DJ, Bergman W, Welvaart K, Scheffer E, van Vloten WA, Russo C, Ferrone S (1984) Immunohistochemical analysis of malignant melanomas and nevocellular nevi with monoclonal antibodies to distinct monomorphic determinants of HLA antigens. Cancer Res 44:3930–3935
Sarna VK, Lundin KEA, Morkrid L, Qiao SW, Sollid LM, Christophersen A (2018) HLA-DQ-Gluten Tetramer blood test accurately identifies patients with and without celiac disease in absence of gluten consumption. Gastroenterology 154(4):886–896
Spier CM, Grogan TM, Lippman SM, Slymen DJ, Rybski JA, Miller TP (1988) The aberrancy of immunophenotype and immunoglobuline status as indicators of prognosis in B-cell difuse large-cell lymphoma. Am J Pathol 133:118–126
Stamnaes I, Sollid LM (2015) Celiac disease: autoimmunity in response to food antigen. Semin Immunol 27(5):343–352
Stimac E, Urieli-Shoval S, Kempin S, Pious D (1991) Defective HLA- DRA X box binding in the class II trans activator transcription factor mutant 6.1.6 and in cell lines from class II immunedeficient patients. J Immunol 146:4398–4405
Taramelli D, Fosati G, Mazzochi A, Delia D, Ferrone S, Parmiani G (1986) Class I and II HLA and melanoma associated antigen expression and modulation on melanoma cells isolated from primary and metastatic lesions. Cancer Res 46:433–439
Van Duinen SG, Mauw BJ, de Graaff-Reitsma CB, Ruiter DJ (1984) Methods in laboratory investigation: Immunoelectron microscopic methods for demonstration of antigens on normal human melanocytes and other epidermal cells. Lab Invest 50:733–741
Wang E, Worschech A, Marincola FM (2008) The immunological constant of rejection. Trends Immunol 29:256–262
Wilson BS, Indiveri F, Pellegrino MA, Ferrone S (1979) DR (Ia-like) antigens on human melanoma cells. Serological detection and immunohistochemical characterization. J Exp Med 149:658–668
Zaloudik J, Moore M, Ghosh AK, Mechl Z, Rejthar A (1988) DNA content and MHC class II antigen expression in malignant melanoma: clinical course. J Clin Pathol 41:1078–1084

Looking into the Future

The restoration of the HLA class I mediated antigen presentation in tumor cells is essential. It allows T lymphocytes to recover the recognition and the rejection of tumors. As indicated several times in this book, the concept of "Hard" versus "Soft" molecular HLA lesions has an enormous implication in the escape or rejection of metastatic lesions during immunotherapy. Current immunotherapies can induce HLA class I upregulation and rejection in metastatic lesions with "Reversible/Soft alterations". Different types of traditional and new generation modern immunotherapy protocols are, in fact, inducing the recovery of HLA-I molecules by modifying the tumor microenviroment and stimulating T cell secretion of Th type 1 cytokines, such as interferons. However, tumor cells with "Irreversible/Hard molecular" HLA alterations represent a real threat to the efficacy of cancer immunotherapy and require gene therapy approach for HLA restoration. Hence, we will need to fight "hard lesions" caused by structural genetic lesions produced by DNA point mutations or micro- or macro-deletions affecting the β2 microglobulin gene or the chromosome region that includes the HLA region, as well as the genetic lesions in the interferon activation pathways. It is a long way before these therapies can be implemented in the clinical setting, but the characterization of these HLA class-I alterations in progressing metastatic lesions resistant to immunotherapy will probably speed up the clinical application of this strategy (Fig. 1).

F. Garrido, *MHC Class-I Loss and Cancer Immune Escape*, Advances in Experimental Medicine and Biology 1151, https://doi.org/10.1007/978-3-030-17864-2

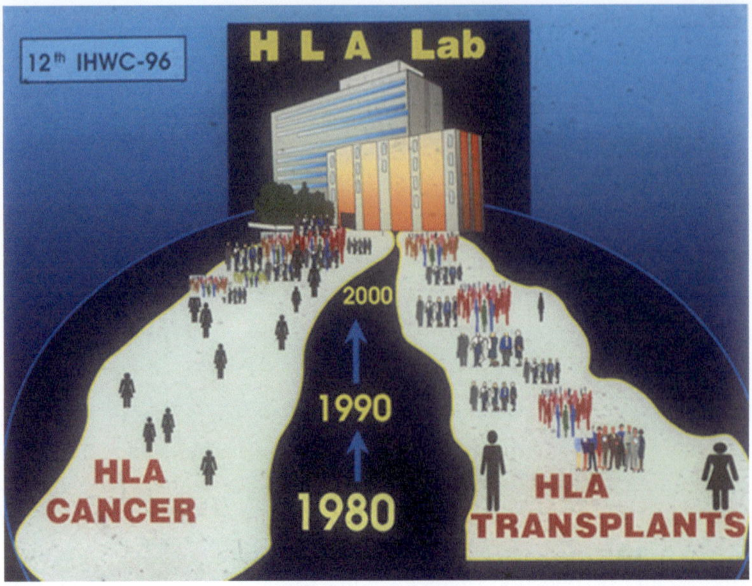

Fig. 1 The relevance of HLA tissue typing in Transplant and Cancer patients. I did this comparison at the 12th International Histocompatibility Workshop and Conference that took place in 1996 in Saint Malo (France) and Paris where the "HLA and Cancer" component was included for the first time. This picture indicates the importance of HLA tissue typing of Cancer patients in our hospitals for the analysis of HLA class I alterations in tumor tissues in order to select a personalized specific treatment as it has been always done for organ transplantation

Concluding Remarks

A Darwinian type of immune selection occurs during tumor development. There are increasing evidences that T lymphocytes are playing a crucial role in recognizing, destroying and rejecting experimental and human tumors. Multiple tumor antigens have been identified that are recognized by T cells as small peptides in the context of the MHC/HLA molecules. At the same time, T cells are selecting HLA-I deficient tumor escape variants that appear in the primary tumor lesion producing at the end a tumor tissue that is composed only of homogeneously HLA-I negative tumor cells. Total or selective losses of HLA class I antigens have been reported in more that 90% of the studied tumours. HLA class I loss is, without any doubt, a major cancer escape mechanism that is frequently observed in tumors originated in different organs. Due to the complexity of the HLA system, different altered tumor phenotypes can be identified in human tumors: HLA I total loss, A,B C locus specific loss, HLA I allelic loss, or HLA haplotype loss. The most important task is to identify and characterize the underlying molecular mechanisms. The new therapies are using antibodies against checkpoint molecules that unblock anti-tumor T lymphocytes. As observed before with "old" immunotherapies, the new generation therapy is also producing "responders", "non responders" and "mixed responders". There are already clear indications that the recurrent and/or progressing metastatic lesions are harbouring "irreversible"molecular alterations that cause a resistance to cytokine-mediated recovery of HLA class I expression. MHC/HLA class I dowregulation should not be seen as an obstacle for T cell based immunotherapy, but as a crucial step in the natural history of tumour development and in the resistance to immunotherapy. There is a long way to go before we undertand why the same treatment produces different responses in different patients , but, without any doubt, MHC/HLA genes and molecules will be playing a leading role in modern cancer immunotherapy in the years to come.

F. Garrido, *MHC Class-I Loss and Cancer Immune Escape*, Advances in Experimental Medicine and Biology 1151, https://doi.org/10.1007/978-3-030-17864-2

Index

F. Garrido, *MHC Class-I Loss and Cancer Immune Escape*, Advances in Experimental Medicine and Biology 1151, https://doi.org/10.1007/978-3-030-17864-2